Advances in Diagnostic and Therapeutic Techniques in Equine Reproduction

Editor

MARCO A. COUTINHO DA SILVA

VETERINARY CLINICS OF NORTH AMERICA: EQUINE PRACTICE

www.vetequine.theclinics.com

Consulting Editor
THOMAS J. DIVERS

December 2016 • Volume 32 • Number 3

ELSEVIER

1600 John F. Kennedy Boulevard • Suite 1800 • Philadelphia, Pennsylvania, 19103-2899

http://www.vetequine.theclinics.com

VETERINARY CLINICS OF NORTH AMERICA: EQUINE PRACTICE Volume 32, Number 3
December 2016 ISSN 0749-0739, ISBN-13: 978-0-323-47754-3

Editor: Katie Pfaff
Developmental Editor: Donald Mumford

Photocopying

Single photocopies of single articles may be made for personal use as allowed by national copyright laws. Permission of the Publisher and payment of a fee is required for all other photocopying, including multiple or systematic copying, copying for advertising or promotional purposes, resale, and all forms of document delivery. Special rates are available for educational institutions that wish to make photocopies for non-profit educational classroom use. For information on how to seek permission visit www.elsevier.com/permissions or call: (+44) 1865 843830 (UK)/(+1) 215 239 3804 (USA).

Derivative Works

Subscribers may reproduce tables of contents or prepare lists of articles including abstracts for internal circulation within their institutions. Permission of the Publisher is required for resale or distribution outside the institution. Permission of the Publisher is required for all other derivative works, including compilations and translations (please consult www. elsevier.com/permissions).

Electronic Storage or Usage

Permission of the Publisher is required to store or use electronically any material contained in this periodical, including any article or part of an article (please consult www.elsevier.com/permissions). Except as outlined above, no part of this publication may be reproduced, stored in a retrieval system or transmitted in any form or by any means, electronic, mechanical, photocopying, recording or otherwise, without prior written permission of the Publisher.

Notice

No responsibility is assumed by the Publisher for any injury and/or damage to persons or property as a matter of products liability, negligence or otherwise, or from any use or operation of any methods, products, instructions or ideas contained in the material herein. Because of rapid advances in the medical sciences, in particular, independent verification of diagnoses and drug dosages should be made.

Although all advertising material is expected to conform to ethical (medical) standards, inclusion in this publication does not constitute a guarantee or endorsement of the quality or value of such product or of the claims made of it by its manufacturer.

Veterinary Clinics of North America: Equine Practice (ISSN 0749-0739) is published in April, August, and December by Elsevier Inc., 360 Park Avenue South, New York, NY 10010-1710. Business and Editorial Offices: 1600 John F. Kennedy Blvd., Suite 1800, Philadelphia, PA 19103-2899. Subscription prices are $270.00 per year (domestic individuals), $477.00 per year (domestic institutions), $100.00 per year (domestic students/residents), $315.00 per year (Canadian individuals), $601.00 per year (Canadian institutions), $365.00 per year (international individuals), $601.00 per year (international institutions), and $180.00 per year (international and Canadian students/residents). To receive student/resident rate, orders must be accompanied by name of affiliated institution, date of term, and the signature of program/residency coordinator on institution letterhead. Orders will be billed at individual rate until proof of status is received. Foreign air speed delivery is included in all *Clinics* subscription prices. All prices are subject to change without notice. **POSTMASTER:** Send address changes to *Veterinary Clinics of North America: Equine Practice*, 3251 Riverport Lane, Maryland Heights, MO 63043. Customer Service (orders, claims, online, change of address): Elsevier Health Sciences Division, Subscription **Customer Service, 3251 Riverport Lane, Maryland Heights, MO 63043. Tel: 1-800-654-2452 (U.S. and Canada); 314-447-8871 (outside U.S. and Canada). Fax: 314-447-8029. E-mail: journalscustomerservice-usa@elsevier.com (for print support);** E-mail: **journalsonlinesupport-usa@elsevier. com (for online support)**.

Reprints. For copies of 100 or more of articles in this publication, please contact the Commercial Reprints Department, Elsevier Inc., 360 Park Avenue South, New York, NY 10010-1710. Tel.: 212-633-3874; Fax: 212-633-3820; E-mail: reprints@elsevier.com.

Veterinary Clinics of North America: Equine Practice is covered in *MEDLINE/PubMed (Index Medicus), Excerpta Medica, Current Contents/Agriculture, Biology and Environmental Sciences,* and *ISI*.

Contributors

CONSULTING EDITOR

THOMAS J. DIVERS, DVM
Diplomate, American College of Veterinary Internal Medicine; Diplomate, American College of Veterinary Emergency and Critical Care; Steffen Professor of Veterinary Medicine, Section Chief, Section of Large Animal Medicine, College of Veterinary Medicine, Cornell University, Ithaca, New York

EDITOR

MARCO A. COUTINHO DA SILVA, DVM, MSc, PhD
Diplomate, American College of Theriogenologists; Clinical Associate Professor, Department of Veterinary Clinical Sciences, The Ohio State University, College of Veterinary Medicine, Columbus, Ohio

AUTHORS

MARCO ANTONIO ALVARENGA, DVM, PhD
Department of Animal Reproduction and Veterinary Radiology, São Paulo State University—UNESP, Botucatu, Brazil

BARRY A. BALL, DVM, PhD
Diplomate, American College of Theriogenologists; Professor and Albert G. Clay Endowed Chair in Equine Reproduction, Department of Veterinary Science, Gluck Equine Research Center, University of Kentucky, Lexington, Kentucky

TERESA A. BURNS, DVM, PhD
Diplomate, American College of Veterinary Internal Medicine (Large Animal); Clinical Assistant Professor, Equine Internal Medicine, The Ohio State University, College of Veterinary Medicine, Columbus, Ohio

IGOR F. CANISSO, DVM, MSc, PhD
Assistant Professor, Department of Veterinary Clinical Medicine, College of Veterinary Medicine, University of Illinois Urbana-Champaign, Urbana, Illinois

ELAINE M. CARNEVALE, DVM, MS, PhD
Professor, Equine Reproduction Laboratory, Department of Biomedical Sciences, Colorado State University, Fort Collins, Colorado

YOUNG-HO CHOI, DVM, PhD
Diplomate, American College of Theriogenologists; Research Associate Professor, Department of Veterinary Physiology and Pharmacology, College of Veterinary Medicine & Biomedical Sciences, Texas A&M University, College Station, Texas

ANTHONY N.J. CLAES, DVM, PhD
Diplomate, American College of Theriogenologists; Assistant Professor in Equine Reproduction, Department of Equine Science, Faculty of Veterinary Medicine, Utrecht University, Utrecht, The Netherlands

MARCO A. COUTINHO DA SILVA, DVM, MSc, PhD
Diplomate, American College of Theriogenologists; Clinical Associate Professor, Department of Veterinary Clinical Sciences, The Ohio State University, College of Veterinary Medicine, Columbus, Ohio

RYAN A. FERRIS, DVM, MS
Diplomate, American College of Theriogenologists; Assistant Professor, Equine Reproduction Laboratory, Department of Clinical Sciences, Colorado State University, Fort Collins, Colorado

KATRIN HINRICHS, DVM, PhD
Diplomate, American College of Theriogenologists; Professor, Department of Veterinary Physiology and Pharmacology, College of Veterinary Medicine & Biomedical Sciences, Texas A&M University, College Station, Texas

CHARLES C. LOVE, DVM, PhD
Diplomate, American College of Theriogenologists; Professor, Section of Theriogenology, Department of Large Animal Clinical Sciences, College of Veterinary Medicine, Texas A&M University, College Station, Texas

PATRICK M. McCUE, DVM, PhD
Diplomate, American College of Theriogenologists; Equine Reproduction Laboratory, College of Veterinary Medicine and Biomedical Sciences, Colorado State University, Fort Collins, Colorado

SUE M. McDONNELL, MA, PhD
Adjunct Professor, New Bolton Center, University of Pennsylvania School of Veterinary Medicine, Kennett Square, Pennsylvania

FREDERICO OZANAM PAPA, DVM, PhD
Department of Animal Reproduction and Veterinary Radiology, São Paulo State University—UNESP, Botucatu, Brazil

KINDRA RADER, BS
Clinical ICSI Program Coordinator, Department of Veterinary Physiology and Pharmacology, College of Veterinary Medicine & Biomedical Sciences, Texas A&M University, College Station, Texas

CARLOS RAMIRES NETO, DVM, MS
Department of Animal Reproduction and Veterinary Radiology, São Paulo State University—UNESP, Botucatu, Brazil

CHARLES F. SCOGGIN, DVM, MS
Diplomate, American College of Theriogenologists; LeBlanc Reproduction Center, Rood and Riddle Equine Hospital, Lexington, Kentucky

EDWARD L. SQUIRES, MS, PhD, ACT (hon)
Professor, Department of Veterinary Science, Maxwell H. Gluck Equine Research Center, University of Kentucky, Lexington, Kentucky

JAMIE STEWART, DVM, MS
Department of Veterinary Clinical Medicine, College of Veterinary Medicine, University of Illinois Urbana-Champaign, Urbana, Illinois

DICKSON D. VARNER, DVM, MS
Diplomate, American College of Theriogenologists; Professor and Pin Oak Stud Chair of Stallion Reproductive Studies, Department of Large Animal Clinical Sciences, College of Veterinary Medicine & Biomedical Sciences, Texas A&M University, College Station, Texas

Contents

Assisted Reproduction

Elaine M. Carnevale

Assisted reproductive techniques that are based on oocyte manipulations
have gained acceptance in the equine industry. Methods to collect and
handle immature or maturing oocytes have been developed, and systems
to ship oocytes now allow for collection in one location and intracytoplasmic sperm injection (ICSI) in another. Subsequently, ICSI-produced
embryos can be transferred onsite, shipped to another location, or cryopreserved. Methods for the collection, identification, culture, maturation,
and shipment of equine oocytes are reviewed, with an emphasis on procedures from laboratories providing clinical services with documented
success.

Kindra Rader, Young-Ho Choi, and Katrin Hinrichs

Intracytoplasmic sperm injection is becoming a common clinical procedure in the horse, but little information is available on techniques for its performance. Each laboratory uses different procedures and different media
for the steps involved with in vitro embryo production. This article outlines
the procedures used in the Clinical Equine Intracytoplasmic Sperm Injection Program at Texas A&M University for in vitro blastocyst production
during the past 3 years.

Edward L. Squires

Most equine embryos are collected from the donor mare and transferred
immediately as fresh embryos or shipped cooled to a recipient station
for transfer within 24 hours. Very few equine embryos are frozen despite
the numerous advantages of embryo cryopreservation. There are 2 major
hurdles: Only the small embryos (<300 μm) provide good pregnancy rates
after freezing/thawing and transfer. Also there is no good procedure for
superovulating mares; thus, extra embryos for freezing are not readily
available. Using either a slow cool or a vitrification method, pregnancy
rates of small equine embryos after freezing/thawing are 50% to 70%.

Endocrinology

Non-Pregnant Mare

categories within breeding seasons or estrous cycles or may fit in multiple classifications. This chapter will focus on discussing etiology and management strategies for mares affected by persistent post-breeding endometritis. Overall, these mares are considered subfertile but acceptable pregnancy and foaling rates can be achieved with appropriate breeding management.

Ryan A. Ferris

Infectious endometritis is among the leading causes of subfertility in the mare. However, the best way to reliably diagnose these cases of infectious endometritis can be confusing to the veterinary practitioner. The goal of this article is to describe how to perform various sample collection techniques, what analyses can be performed on these samples, and how to interpret the results of these analysis. Additionally, future technologies will be presented that are not currently used in equine reproduction practice.

Charles F. Scoggin

Endometritis is characterized by inflammation of the endometrial lining of the uterus and is a leading cause of subfertility in broodmares. When traditional therapies fall short, nonconventional means can be used either to supplement or in lieu of customary practices to manage endometritis. This article reviews alternative therapies available for use in broodmare practice and provides anecdotal and scientific evidence supporting their use.

Stallion

Sue M. McDonnell

Despite the suboptimal aspects of domestic breeding conditions compared with the natural conditions under which their reproductive behavior evolved, most domestic stallions can adapt to management and breeding programs. Most respond adequately or quickly learn to safely abide the restraint and direction of a human handler, and can adapt to changes in methods of breeding for semen collection. If not, the problems can range from inadequate or variable sexual interest and response to overenthusiastic or aggressive response beyond the ability of the handlers to safely direct and control. This article discusses veterinary evaluation as well as housing and handling strategies for addressing stallion breeding behavior problems.

Marco Antonio Alvarenga, Frederico Ozanam Papa, and Carlos Ramires Neto

The use of stallion frozen semen minimizes the spread of disease, eliminates geographic barriers, and preserves the genetic material of the animal for an unlimited time. Significant progress on the frozen thawed stallion semen process and consequent fertility has been achieved over the last decade. These improvements not only increased fertility rates but also allowed cryopreservation of semen from "poor freezers." This article reviews traditional steps and new strategies for stallion semen handling and processing that are performed to overcome the deleterious effects of semen preservation and consequently improve frozen semen quality and fertility.

Stallion semen evaluation is an important part of the breeding soundness evaluation. The results of the semen evaluation cannot be interpreted without a thorough knowledge of the mare and management effects that may have played a role or may affect the potential fertility of the stallion evaluated. There are considerations and limitations that the clinician should understand about each test. Any sperm quality test must be interpreted with a clear understanding of how it relates to fertility.

Subfertility can be a confusing term because some semen of good quality can have reduced fertility following cooled transport if the semen is processed in an improper manner. General procedures aimed at processing stallion semen for cooled transport are well described. An array of factors could exist in reduced fertility of cool-transported semen. This article focuses on centrifugation techniques that can be used to maximize sperm quality of stallions whose semen is intended for cooled transport. Clinical cases are also provided for practical application of techniques.

VETERINARY CLINICS OF
NORTH AMERICA: EQUINE PRACTICE

THE CLINICS ARE NOW AVAILABLE ONLINE!
Access your subscription at:
www.theclinics.com

Preface

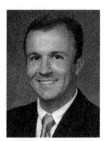

Marco A. Coutinho da Silva, DVM, MSc, PhD, DACT
Editor

It has been 10 years since the last issue of *Veterinary Clinics of North America: Equine Practice* focused on equine reproduction. During this decade, there has been remarkable progress on our understanding of many physiologic and pathologic processes, leading to new and alternative therapies for many reproductive conditions. The purpose of this issue is to highlight these state-of-the-art techniques and concepts that are currently being applied in equine practice. Each article was designed to contain relevant scientific information on the topic while remaining practical and informative.

I am fortunate to have been invited to serve as guest editor of this issue and could not have accomplished this project without the collaboration of my colleagues and mentors that participated in this issue. They are experts in their field of study and have been generous in providing such invaluable content.

Appreciatively,

Marco A. Coutinho da Silva, DVM, MSc, PhD, DACT
Department of Veterinary Clinical Sciences
College of Veterinary Medicine
The Ohio State University
Columbus, OH 43210, USA

E-mail address:
coutinho-da-silva.1@osu.edu

Vet Clin Equine 32 (2016) xiii
http://dx.doi.org/10.1016/j.cveq.2016.09.001
0749-0739/16/© 2016 Published by Elsevier Inc.

vetequine.theclinics.com

Advances in Collection, Transport and Maturation of Equine Oocytes for Assisted Reproductive Techniques

Elaine M. Carnevale, DVM, MS, PhD

KEYWORDS

- Equine • Oocyte • Maturation • Collection • Assisted reproduction
- Intracytoplasmic sperm injection • Culture

KEY POINTS

- Oocytes can be collected from harvested ovaries or from live mares for assisted fertilization using intracytoplasmic sperm injection.
- Oocytes can be collected from immature follicles or follicles that have been induced to mature by the administration of ovulation-inducing compounds to the donor mare.
- The appearance of follicle cells surrounding the oocyte are indicative of state of maturation or atresia.
- Ovaries and oocytes can be shipped to central facilities for intracytoplasmic sperm injection.

INTRODUCTION

Assisted reproductive techniques that are based on oocyte manipulations have gained acceptance in the equine industry. Methods to collect and handle immature or maturing oocytes have been developed, and systems to ship oocytes now allow for collection in one location and intracytoplasmic sperm injection (ICSI) in another. Subsequently, ICSI-produced embryos can be transferred onsite, shipped to another location, or cryopreserved. These advances have increased the use of equine assisted fertilization (ICSI) for stallions with limited quantities or quality of sperm or for subfertile mares. Methods for the collection, identification, culture, maturation, and shipment of equine oocytes are reviewed, with an emphasis on procedures from laboratories providing clinical services with documented success.

Equine Reproduction Laboratory, Department of Biomedical Sciences, Colorado State University, 3101 Rampart Road, Fort Collins, CO 80523-1693, USA
E-mail address: emc@colostate.edu

Vet Clin Equine 32 (2016) 379–399
http://dx.doi.org/10.1016/j.cveq.2016.07.002
0749-0739/16/© 2016 Elsevier Inc. All rights reserved.

OOCYTE COLLECTIONS

In general, oocytes can be collected from 2 types of follicles. Maturing follicles are follicles that have started the process of follicular and oocyte maturation; maturation can be initiated and timed through the administration of ovulation-inducing compounds or naturally with endogenous luteinizing hormone. Immature follicles are follicles that have not been stimulated to mature or are not capable of responding to ovulatory stimuli; they basically include most follicles, with the exception of maturing follicles that are destined to ovulate. Methods to collect equine oocytes from maturing or immature follicles have been developed to accommodate the large size of the maturing follicle during estrus and the strong attachments of immature cumulus oocyte complexes to the follicular wall. Equine oocytes are primarily collected through transvaginal, ultrasound-guided follicle aspirations. Many of the general procedures are similar when collecting oocytes regardless of the follicle type.

SEDATION AND ANALGESIA

Proper preparation and sedation of the donor mare are essential for oocyte collections. We administer flunixin meglumine (300–500 mg) within 15 minutes before oocyte collection, although some laboratories will administer flunixin meglumine directly after immature oocyte collections.[1] In general, flunixin meglumine seems to have a marginal effect on the mare's comfort during the procedure; however, it does reduce the incidence of mild colic after oocyte collections, which is uncommon but observed more often after small follicle aspirations than maturing follicle aspirations. In nervous mares or mares with a "tight" reproductive tract, acepromazine (10–20 mg) can be administered intramuscularly at the time of flunixin meglumine administration to assist relaxation. Because acepromazine relaxes the posterior reproductive tract, it will increase the chance of pneumovagina in some mares. Just before the procedure, N-butylscopolammonium (100–150 mg) is administered to prevent rectal contractions. Sedation and analgesia can be provided with a combination of butorphanol (5–10 mg) and xylazine hydrochloride (150–400 mg) or detomidine hydrochloride (2–5 mg). For most mares, xylazine provides adequate sedation for the short duration of a maturing oocyte collection, and additional xylazine can be administered if the mare is moving or uncomfortable during the procedure. For fractious or nervous mares, a low dose of detomidine (2–3 mg) can be administered in the stall before the mare entering the stocks, with xylazine (100–300 mg) administered just before the oocyte collection. As a subjective observation, xylazine seems to reduce discomfort associated with manipulation of the maturing follicle to a greater extent than detomidine. However, for the longer interval of sedation required for small follicle aspirations, repeated doses of detomidine (4–6 mg) are often used. To provide the best sedation, we modify our regime for individual mares and log the compounds and results; this allows us to have an optimal and repeatable regime specific to each mare. Although sedation varies, we consistently administer N-butylscopolammonium, butorphanol, and flunixin meglumine for aspirations, and for shorter procedures, mares are twitched.

GENERAL PROCEDURES FOR OOCYTE COLLECTIONS

Before beginning the oocyte collection, all equipment, supplies, and media should be prepared and warmed as needed. Different needle systems have been used to collect oocytes, but most involve a 12-gauge, double-lumen needle attached to a suction pump and collection bottle, with a method to inject flush medium into the follicles. Needles for oocyte collections are commercially available (Mila International, Inc,

Florence, KY; Minitube of America, Inc, Verona, WI); the double lumen allows flush to be injected into the follicle simultaneously or alternately with suction of follicular contents. Tubing runs in and out of a sterile collection bottle allowing the aspiration pump to assert negative pressure at approximately 150 mm Hg; however, the collection flow rate can vary with tubing length and needle configuration, and suction can be adjusted accordingly. Lower suction is often used when follicles are alternately being filled and suctioned, as with immature follicles, to allow the follicles to properly fill with flush solution.

Various media have been used to lavage follicles during oocyte collections, with the most common being sterile, packaged embryo flush solutions[2,3] or Medium 199 with Hank salts, HEPES, gentamycin, and 0.4% fetal bovine serum.[1] Heparin (5–20 IU/mL) is added to the medium to prevent coagulation. Commercial flush media are also available that are specifically marketed for oocyte collections. Media should be maintained at approximately body temperature, particularly when maturing oocytes are being collected. Tubing is available with a T-connection (Controlled Flushing Set; Mila International, Inc), which allows medium to be pulled directly from the bag or from sterile bottle into an injection syringe and then discharged into the tubing attached to the needle. As an alternative, media can be pulled into all-plastic syringes and injected directly into the needle tubing.

When equipment and media are ready, the mare is placed within stocks, and her tail is wrapped and tied. We do an initial cleaning of the perineal area, before inserting a few squares of gauze within the vestibule. The gauze helps to prevent lube, water, or manure from entering the vestibule, especially if the mare has poor perineal conformation or has been given a sedative. The rectum is then cleaned of manure. If excess air is present in the rectum, a dose syringe attached to y-tubing or another device to provide gentle suction can be used to help with its evacuation. After this, the perineal area is thoroughly scrubbed, and the gauze squares are removed.

For aspirations, an ultrasound transducer is housed in a casing with a needle guide. A sterile, nontoxic lube is placed on the transducer face, and a sleeve or other sheath can be used to cover the transducer. Additional lube can then be applied to the probe and casing. The transducer is placed in the anterior vagina without allowing air to enter, as the air can impair contact between the vaginal wall and transducer face and cause imaging problems. If air is present in the vagina, gentle downward pressure on the rectum dorsal to the anterior vagina can help to evacuate it. The transducer is positioned lateral to the cervix on the side ipsilateral to the ovary to be aspirated. The location of the transducer in relation to the cervix can be confirmed through rectal palpation before positioning the ovary. The ovary should be flipped to the medial side of the broad ligament before being brought posterior to the face of the transducer. The surface of the ovary can be palpated to help determine optimal positioning and to ensure that no structures, other than the vaginal and follicular walls, are between the ovary and end of the needle guide. During the ovarian puncture and aspiration, the ovary should be held firmly without irritating or damaging the rectum.

OOCYTE COLLECTION FROM MATURING DOMINANT FOLLICLES

Accurate timing of oocyte maturation is important when collecting oocytes from maturing follicles. Therefore, induction compounds must be administered when the follicle is capable of responding to the stimuli but before the endogenous initiation of follicle maturation. General criteria for administration of maturation-inducing compounds are a follicle at least 33 mm in diameter and endometrial edema. This should be associated with an estrous mare and/or relaxation of uterine and cervical tone consistent with estrus and the follicular phase. Maturation criteria can vary for individual mares, with some mares maturing larger or smaller follicles. Follicle maturation is induced through the administration of human chorionic gonadotropin or a gonadotropin-releasing hormone analog, such as deslorelin acetate, or a combination of both. The maturing oocyte is often collected 20 to 24 hours after administration of induction compounds. However, oocytes can be collected until the approximate time of ovulation, estimated at 36 to 40 hours after induction.

The collection of an oocyte from the dominant, maturing follicle has the benefit of an oocyte that has started the maturation process in vivo, and further stimulation of oocyte maturation is not required in vitro. Only 1 or 2 follicles will usually respond to maturation induction during a mare's estrous cycle. At the same time, oocytes can be collected from secondary follicles. Oocytes from the secondary follicles are typically immature and often in some stage of atresia; these oocytes will require hormonal stimulation in vitro and additional time for the completion of maturation.

For collection of the maturing oocyte, the follicle is positioned to ensure that the oviduct, ovulation fossa, and broad ligament are not punctured with the needle. Other than the apex of the follicle, ovarian stroma should not be punctured. The needle is advanced well into the antrum to prevent the follicle wall from collapsing away from the bevel as follicular fluid is removed. As the follicle and oocyte approach maturation and ovulation, the oocyte can be more easily dislodged from the follicle; however, damage to the oocyte, for example, fracture of the zona pellucida, is more likely to occur especially if suction pressure is high (**Fig. 1**). When collecting maturing oocytes in our laboratory, a gentle flow of flush medium is maintained while manually collapsing the follicle wall toward the needle shaft. The needle is moved to different areas within the follicle, and the bevel is intermittently turned. In other laboratories, the follicle is filled with flush and collapsed at least 10 times, while massaging and balloting the follicle per rectum.[3] For a typical maturing follicle, the aspirate will initially be golden yellow as follicular fluid is removed. However, as the highly vascular follicle wall is disrupted, the aspirate will become bloody, and sheets of mucoid granulosa cells can be observed floating within the aspirate.

The maturing oocyte is sensitive to temperature changes; therefore, media, plastic ware, and all contacting surfaces should be warmed to approximately body temperature. Heating plates and stage warmers are helpful to prevent temperature variations

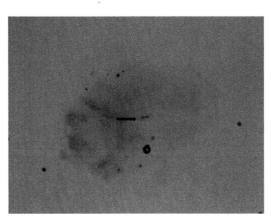

Fig. 1. Maturing cumulus oocyte complex with a damaged oocyte after the zona pellucida was fractured; note the dispersed and elongated ooplasm (*arrow*).

while searching for oocytes. The aspirate should not be filtered, as maturing granulosa cells are mucoid and will clog the filter. We pour the aspirate into multiple large (150 × 25 mm) polystyrene Petri dishes to search for the cumulus oocyte complex (**Fig. 2**). For most aspirations, a large number of granulosa cells will be present in the aspirate, and granulosa cells can be attached to the cumulus oocyte complex (see **Fig. 2**). The cumulus cells that surround the oocyte have a fine texture, and they are typically clear or slightly yellow in appearance (**Fig. 3**). The intact cumulus oocyte complex expands into the follicle, with a ring of tighter cells (corona radiata) encircling the oocyte (**Fig. 4**). The maturing cumulus oocyte complex can often be identified by gross observation of the aspirate (**Fig. 5**). If the cumulus complex is not identified, the aspirate needs to be carefully searched for the oocyte, which can be stripped from part of the cumulus complex (**Fig. 6**). On identification, the oocyte is quickly washed to remove blood before it is placed into culture. In our laboratory, Tissue Culture Medium 199 with Hank salts and additions of 10% fetal calf serum and 25 μg/mL gentamicin is used as a wash; Hank salts help to buffer the medium for room atmosphere. The oocyte flush medium or an embryo-holding medium also can be used to rinse the cumulus oocyte complex. For the large, sticky cumulus oocyte complexes associated with maturing oocytes, a 0.25-mL, gamma-irradiated straw can be attached to a ureteral catheter connector and 1-mL syringe to move it between solutions. Preferably, the complex is slowly pulled into the straw from the attached granulosa cells to avoid excess tension on the oocyte (**Fig. 7A**). On occasion, the cumulus oocyte complex is very large because of the associated granulosa cells. In those cases, some of the granulosa cells should be removed before trying to move the complex. This is best done by positioning two 21-gauge or 23-gauge needles so that the tips cross and cut through the cells (**Fig. 7B**).

An oocyte can be collected from more than 70% of maturing follicles with training,[2–4] and rates can be higher with additional experience. In general, only 1 or 2 maturing follicles are available during a cycle. Although administration of a low dose of equine follicle-stimulating hormone (eFSH) increased the maturing follicle numbers and recovered oocytes per cycle,[4] no recombinant compound or viable alternative is commercially available at this time. When obtained from the maturing follicle and cultured under appropriate conditions, nearly all oocytes from normal follicles mature to metaphase II, as judged by extrusion of a polar body.[3,4] In our clinical and

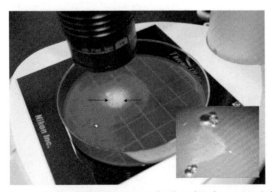

Fig. 2. Aspirates from maturing follicles are searched within large Petri dishes. The bloody appearance is normal, as the vascular network surrounding the follicle is disrupted during the aspiration. A sheet of expanded granulosa cells is imaged (*black arrows*), and the cumulus oocyte complex (*white arrows*) is attached to more granulosa cells.

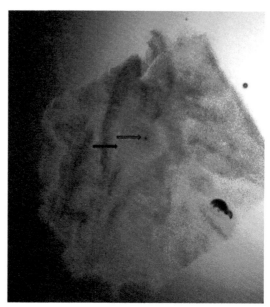

Fig. 3. A maturing cumulus oocyte complex, with surrounding granulosa cells, expanding cumulus cells (*dark arrow*), and an oocyte (*clear arrow*).

research ICSI programs, it is rare to have oocytes from maturing follicles that do not extrude a polar body, and most of these are associated with specific problem mares.

OOCYTE COLLECTION FROM IMMATURE FOLLICLES

Oocyte collections can be attempted from the entire population of antral follicles, with most laboratories aspirating all follicles larger than 5 to 10 mm in diameter.[5–7] The oocytes within these follicles are typically immature or in some stage of atresia. Collections of immature oocytes can be done on a timed schedule, regardless of cycle, with

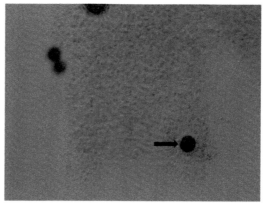

Fig. 4. Cumulus complex in which some of the cells have torn off, exposing the oocyte (*arrow*) and the surrounding corona radiata. The oocyte is often difficult to image this clearly because of the surrounding cumulus cells.

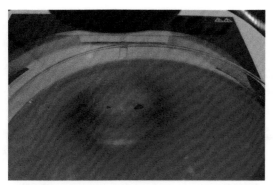

Fig. 5. Mature cumulus cells within the aspirate have a distinct clear appearance. Note the more granular sheets of granulosa cells within the aspirate.

10 to 14 days between aspiration attempts to allow growth of a new wave of follicles before the subsequent aspiration,[5,7] although criteria of at least 5 follicles larger than 5 mm have been established before aspiration.[5] Donors can also be monitored with ultrasonography to optimize the time of oocyte collection. This is done with some older, problem mares, ensuring at least 8 follicles larger than 10 mm are present at the time of aspiration.[6]

The cumulus oocyte complex is firmly attached to the follicular wall in immature equine follicles.[8] This broad and complex attachment makes removal of the oocyte more difficult than from the follicles of other species or from the maturing equine follicle (**Fig. 8**). Simple puncture and aspiration of fluid from immature follicles in the mare results in low oocyte recovery; therefore, methods have been developed to help dislodge the equine oocyte from the follicle to improve collection rates. The donor mare is prepared for oocyte collections similar to maturing follicle aspirations, with the exception that the bladder can be catheterized to prevent its enlargement, which can affect probe positioning and/or urination during the procedure. The ovary is positioned per rectum to allow the clinician or an assistant to puncture single follicles or move through a series of follicles within the ovarian stroma. After each puncture,

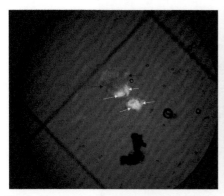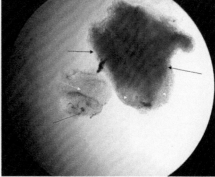

Fig. 6. The cumulus oocyte complex has been torn apart with a section of cumulus cells (*white arrows*) containing the oocyte (*red arrow in enlarged image*); additional cumulus cells (*white arrows*) are attached to a sheet of granulosa cells (*black arrows*) in the bloody aspirate and wash dish under higher magnification.

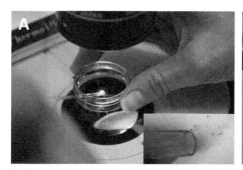
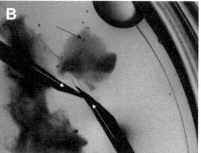

Fig. 7. A cumulus oocyte complex is being transferred into wash medium using a 0.25-mL straw (*A*); the insert shows image as seen through a stereoscope. The tips of 2 needles (*white arrows*) being used to trim a large sheet of granulosa cells (left of needles) from the cumulus oocyte (*dark arrow*) complex (*B*).

follicular fluid is aspirated before inflation of the follicle with a flush medium. This is repeated, while the needle is rapidly rotated back and forth during the aspiration phase. The process is repeated approximately 6 times per follicle.[1] The needle is then moved into an adjacent follicle, and the procedure is repeated. For the collection of oocytes from limited or larger subordinate follicles, the clinician can collapse and massage the follicular wall over the shaft and bevel of the needle with gentle rotation of the needle. When small follicle aspirations are complete, the aspirate can be run through an embryo collection filter with a 75-μm mesh; the filter is thoroughly rinsed, and the aspirate is searched for oocytes (**Fig. 9**).

The number of oocytes that can be collected per immature follicle aspiration session varies with number of ovarian follicles and techniques. Oocyte collection rates have improved over time as better methods have been developed for the mare. Although historical oocyte collection rates were often less than 50% per immature follicle, rates of 50% to 70% have now been reported,[6,7] with 4 to 12 oocytes per mare per

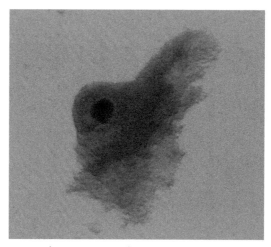

Fig. 8. The immature cumulus oocyte complex is attached to the follicular wall and associated granulosa cells in a broad-based hillock, making removal from the follicle difficult.

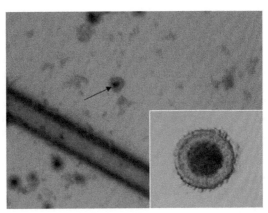

Fig. 9. Immature granulosa cells and oocyte (*arrow*) within a search dish and enlarged image (*insert*) of an immature oocyte with a tight ring of surrounding corona cells.

collection session.[3,6,7,9] However, success will vary with the individual mare and technical experience of the collection unit. The collection of oocytes from small follicles has advantages of scheduled aspiration times and potential to collect numerous oocytes per aspiration session. In contrast to maturing oocytes, immature oocytes are less temperature sensitive and provide more flexibility for timing shipments, maturation, and ICSI. Not all immature oocytes will successfully complete maturation in vitro, with reported maturation rates of 50% to 88% per oocyte,[3,6,7,9] although the highest maturation rates (up to 88%) were obtained from immature oocytes collected from subordinate follicles, 6 to 30 mm, during the same session as a maturing oocyte.[3] When compared with oocyte collections from maturing follicles, the lower oocyte collection and maturation rates for oocytes from immature/small follicles is offset by the potential to collect more oocytes from numerous follicles.

CLINICAL PROBLEMS ASSOCIATED WITH OOCYTE COLLECTIONS

Few medical problems have been associated with oocyte collections in horses; however, this does not imply that these are innocuous procedures, without any potential risk to the mare. These risks could be considered medical and structural in nature. Medical problems after oocyte collections are not common, but they have been reported and include hemorrhage, peritonitis, colic, rectal bleeding, and ovarian abscesses.[10–13] Therefore, oocyte collections from client mares should be done with caution and after adequate practice or training. Because the needle is puncturing within the abdominal cavity and ovary, the need for maintaining a clean environment is essential, and equipment, supplies, and media must be appropriately cleaned or sterilized.

Mares susceptible to uterine infections or other reproductive problems, such as pneumovagina or urine pooling, can have potential contaminates or irritants within the vagina, and these can be carried into the abdomen with the aspiration needle. If the mare has clinical signs or a history of uterine infections, the uterus can be cultured and treated before oocyte collections. Most mares will not have subsequent uterine infections if care is taken not to introduce additional challenges to the uterus. In mares with fibrotic cervixes or cervical adhesions and mostly anechoic intrauterine fluid, uterine culture procedures could introduce bacteria into susceptible uteri. In these mares, we will often culture the anterior vagina during early estrus to ensure that no gross contamination is present. The vagina also can be lavaged with lactated Ringer solution or saline, with or without antibiotics, before the aspiration procedure.

In some cases, transvaginal procedures for oocyte collections can be difficult or risky for the mare. These could include problems such as recurrent uterine infections with discharge, rectovaginal fistulas, or severe perineal melanomas. In these cases, oocytes can be collected from maturing follicles through the flank. Briefly, a cannula is inserted through the abdominal muscles of the flank, and the ovary is manipulated per rectum to position the large follicle at the internal os of the cannula. A needle is inserted through the cannula and into the follicle, and the follicle is drained of follicular fluid with or without lavage of the antrum.[1,14]

The routine use of antibiotics with oocyte collections is probably not necessary, especially if a single follicle is punctured in a normal mare. However, if potential contamination exists from the mare's reproductive tract, numerous follicles are punctured, or other complicating factors occur, the use of systemic antibiotics is advised. Administration of ampicillin (2 mg/kg) and gentamicin (6.6 mg/kg) within 10 minutes before the start of oocyte collections did not affect blastocyst production.[5] However, additional studies have not been conducted to directly examine the effect of systemic antibiotics or other administered compounds on developmental potential of equine oocytes. In our laboratory, we administer ceftiofur sodium in mares as indicated at the time of oocyte collections, or other antibiotics are used that are specific for organisms associated with a previous uterine or vaginal culture. Mares' temperatures are taken daily for 3 days after an aspiration as our standard procedure. Elevated temperatures are rare, but they provide warning of a potential medical problem.

The extent that oocyte collections could result in structural damage to the ovary and potentially affect long-term fertility is still inconclusive. Procedures for oocyte collections initially involved collection of maturing oocytes from dominant follicles and were used primarily for mares that were incapable of producing embryos or a pregnancy.[2,11,15] However, with the collection of oocytes from young, fertile mares for ICSI using limited or poor-quality sperm, future fertility could be impacted if the ovarian stroma, primordial follicle pool, oviduct, or ovulation fossa are damaged. A decline in fertility has not been documented for the limited number of mares that have been inseminated after oocyte collections.[16,17] However, some ovarian changes have been noted with repeated immature follicle collections. After an 8-year period of immature oocyte collections, the ovaries of 4 mares were observed to be firmer in consistency on palpation, presumably because of formation of fibrous tissue within the ovarian stroma.[10] Other complications noted after immature follicle collections were rectal bleeding and ovarian adhesions,[13] thickening of the ovarian serosa,[1] and ovarian abscesses.[10,13] In the studies, histologic evaluations were limited, with only vague mentions of condensed reparative fibrosis[10] and siderocytes[13] within the ovarian stroma.

OOCYTE COLLECTION FROM HARVESTED OVARIES

When a mare dies or is euthanized for medical reasons, oocytes can be harvested from antral follicles in an attempt to produce additional offspring. If the euthanasia can be timed, optimal results will usually be obtained if a large number of small to medium follicles are available for oocyte harvesting. Mares in mid to late diestrus or early estrus will often have a growing wave of follicles with viable oocytes. Mares with few antral follicles present on the ovaries provide a minimal chance of success. In many cases, this can be assessed before euthanasia by ultrasonography of the ovaries. Presently, most clinicians ship the excised ovaries to more specialized facilities for oocyte collection, maturation, and ICSI. However, as practitioners become more familiar with collecting and handling oocytes, the procedure might be more successful if oocytes are collected directly after the ovaries are removed from the mare, and the oocytes are packaged and shipped to another facility for ICSI. When oocytes are to be harvested from ovaries immediately after euthanasia and directly (<30 minutes) placed into maturation in vitro, the ovaries and oocytes should be kept at approximately body temperature (37–38°C). However, ovaries or oocytes to be shipped should be cooled to room temperature.

The most consistent and successful method for the collection of oocytes from excised ovaries involves the scraping of individual follicles.[18] Scraping versus aspiration of follicles results in the collection of significantly more oocytes, more cumulus-enclosed oocytes, and fewer fertilization abnormalities.[19,20] Before oocyte harvesting, the ovaries are rinsed to remove debris and trimmed of excess tissue. Each palpable follicle is sliced open with a scalpel blade, and follicular fluid is drained into a collection dish or a large Petri dish. The follicular cells are then gently scraped from the inner surface of the follicle, using a bone curette appropriate for the size of the follicle (**Fig. 10**). The curette is rinsed between scrapings or dipped into a tube of medium to remove follicular cells. A complete embryo flush or wash medium can be used. Follicle scrapings can be done in individual Petri dishes to determine if the oocyte was collected from each follicle, or the entire aspirate can be combined and filtered before searching. In our laboratory, we typically search by individual follicles and attempt to move all oocytes to rinse and holding medium as soon as possible. When all surface follicles have been processed, the ovary can be sliced open to look for additional follicles. Even follicles as small as 2 to 3 mm are processed. When no additional follicles are observed, the ovaries are sliced into small segments and thoroughly rinsed with medium. The large collection dish with follicular fluid and rinse medium is searched for additional oocytes. If the oocytes are to be shipped to another facility, they can then be rinsed in an appropriate medium and packaged for shipment, as described later in this article.

OOCYTE CULTURE AND MATURATION

When maturation of the oocyte is initiated in vivo through the administration of induction compounds, oocytes should be recovered during the process of oocyte

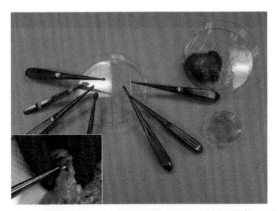

Fig. 10. Bone curettes, scalpel blade, and Petri dishes are prepared for collection of oocytes from harvested ovaries. After follicles are sliced open using a scalpel blade, the follicle cells can be scraped using an appropriately sized bone curette (*insert*).

maturation. In general, at 20 to 24 hours after administration of induction compounds, most oocytes are at or near the metaphase I stage of maturation, with duplicate chromosomes aligned at the metaphase plate. At the time of anticipated ovulation, equine oocytes are typically at metaphase II with extrusion of the first polar body. They are then considered "mature" and ready for fertilization. Therefore, when oocytes are collected after administration of ovulation induction compounds to the donor mare and oocyte maturation is initiated in vivo, no further stimulation of maturation is required in vitro. The maturing oocytes simply can be cultured in medium without the addition of hormones for the completion of the maturation interval.

Different base media have successfully been used for the culture of maturing and immature oocytes, including tissue culture medium 199 (TCM 199),[21] equine maturation medium (EMMI),[22] Dulbecco modified Eagle medium/F12,[23] and combinations of base media.[3] Pyruvate, antibiotics, and serum, albumin, or a serum replacement are often added. Most laboratories culture the oocytes in a humid atmosphere with 5% CO_2 and air, although one laboratory reported culture in 5% CO_2, 5% O_2, and 90% N_2.[3] Incubation temperatures from 37.9 to 38.5°C are currently used.[3,5,24,25] The culture interval until ICSI is usually measured from the administration of induction drugs to the donor mares, with sperm injections performed 40 to 46 hours later.[3,4,7] Therefore, if the oocyte was collected at 24 hours after induction, it would be cultured approximately 18 hours before ICSI. However, the status of the follicle and oocyte should be considered before deciding the timing of ICSI, as some oocytes are close to maturation at the time of collection, and some follicles do not respond to the induction drugs and produce an immature oocyte. If an immature oocyte is collected, based on the morphology of the cumulus and granulosa cells, the oocyte will need to be matured in vitro.

When immature oocytes are matured in vitro, hormones are added to the base media, with the most consistent addition being FSH (5 mU).[3,5,25] However, an array of hormones have been added, including luteinizing hormone (1 μg/mL), FSH (15 ng/mL), estradiol (1 μg/ml), progesterone (200 ng/mL), insulinlike growth factor (10 mg/mL), and epidermal growth factor (100 ng/mL).[26] Oocytes can be cultured under the same atmospheric conditions and temperatures as maturing oocytes. Immature oocytes can be cultured in 0.5 mL of medium in 4-well dishes (Nunc, Roskilde, Denmark) as used in our laboratory[26] or in droplets under oil with 10 μL of medium per oocyte[5] or 4 to 8 oocytes per 30-μL drop.[3] Immature oocytes are typically matured between 24 and 30 hours before ICSI.[3,5,26,27]

OOCYTE IDENTIFICATION

Oocyte identification and assessment are imperative for success, and the practitioner should be familiar with imaging the cumulus oocyte complex.[25,28] In general, oocytes and the associated follicles can be classified as immature, maturing, mature, or atretic. When trying to ascertain the stage of oocyte development, factors other than the visual assessment of oocytes should be considered, including the ultrasound and palpation characteristics of aspirated follicles and cumulus and granulosa cell morphology. Follicles with characteristics consistent with imminent ovulation during palpation (soft and painful) or ultrasonography (thickened follicular wall, irregular shape, rent in wall)[29,30] indicate that the oocyte is close to maturity, even if ovulation induction compounds were not administered. Conversely, follicle maturation is not always successfully induced, and an immature oocyte can be collected from a follicle even after administration of induction drugs. In some cases, large or secondary follicles will undergo atretic changes, which can be detected with ultrasonography as fine echogenic debris within the lumen, loss of vascularity, and no growth or a reduction in size. In addition to follicle characteristics, the cells within the aspirate are important indicators of follicle stage and viability.

The identification of oocytes can be complicated by blood, cellular debris, and surrounding cells. Air bubbles can mimic the appearance of the maturing oocyte when they are trapped under cumulus or granulosa cells. In general, air bubbles have a dark border and clear central area, while the maturing oocytes will have a gray appearance and a ring of cells forming the corona radiata (**Fig. 11**). Immature oocytes have compact cumulus and granulosa cells associated with the oocyte and aspirate; these oocytes are typically at the germinal vesicle stage of maturation (**Fig. 12**). If the donor's dominant follicle did not respond to induction compounds, the oocyte will still be immature. Immature granulosa cells will be present in small sheets of tightly associated cells, in contrast to the loosely arranged and mucoid cells of the mature follicle (**Fig. 13**). Many oocytes from small follicles or secondary follicles will be in some stage of atresia. These follicles will often have cells that appear immature or slightly expanded, although the typical expansion of the preovulatory follicle will not be observed (see **Fig. 13**). Cumulus cells associated with an atretic oocyte can be mottled or clumped in appearance; usually, cells of the corona radiata are still tight. With advanced atresia, the ooplasm can be shrunken, dark, or fragmented (**Fig. 14**).

Cumulus and granulosa cells are markedly changed during the process of maturation in vivo. The cumulus cells surrounding the oocyte begin to expand into a yellowish, clear mass (see **Fig. 3**). When collected just before ovulation, cumulus cells are typically very mucoid and clear (see **Fig. 5**). The corona radiata, which normally appears as a ring of cells around maturing oocytes, continues to expand in a starburst pattern and is less defined. Expansion is also noted in the granulosa cells, with an even, slightly granular appearance. The cells are very mucoid and will string from the dish to straw. When maturation occurs in vitro, the cumulus cells will expand, but they do not obtain the same level of expansion or mucoid nature as when maturation occurs in vivo (see **Fig. 12**).

TRANSPORT OF OVARIES AND OOCYTES
Shipment of Harvested Ovaries

Minimal information has been published on the shipment of equine oocytes, although procedures have already been used for clinical purposes. More substantial

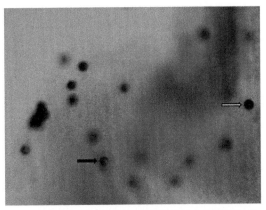

Fig. 11. Oocyte (*dark arrow*), from a maturing follicle, has a dark central area and ring of corona radiata cells; air bubbles (*white arrow*) will be clear with a dark border when in focus. Also note air bubbles in **Figs. 1, 4,** and **13**B.

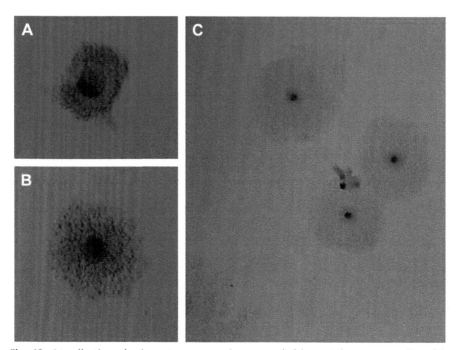

Fig. 12. At collection, the immature oocyte is surrounded by a tight corona radiata (A), which expands in a starburst pattern during maturation (B). After maturation in vitro, immature oocytes will have expanded cumulus cells and a loosening of the cells of the corona radiata (C), but the cumulus complex does not have the massive expansion and mucoid nature characteristic of maturation in vivo.

information has been published regarding the shipping of ovaries and holding of immature oocytes. After death or euthanasia of a mare, ovaries can be shipped to another facility for oocyte collection, maturation, and oocyte transfer or ICSI, with the potential to produce a foal or foals.[27,28,31] The ovaries are removed after death, euthanasia, or surgical anesthesia, rinsed with an embryo flush or physiologic salt solution, and immediately packaged for shipment to the receiving facility. Limited research has been done to determine the optimal temperature for ovary shipment, and most studies conclude at embryo development, but not pregnancies. In one study,[26] ovaries were collected at an abattoir, with no knowledge of mare age or condition. From each mare, one ovary was shipped at approximately 12°C (9–16°C) and the other ovary was shipped at 22°C (12–25°C) with a shipment interval of 18 to 24 hours. Oocytes were matured and multiple oocytes were transferred into inseminated recipients. Of the transferred oocytes, 16% resulted in embryonic vesicles. No difference in pregnancy rates were observed between temperature ranges. The developmental competence of oocytes after ICSI to form blastocysts is impacted by a longer duration of ovary holding (approximately 21 vs 7 hours).[32] In general, refrigeration temperatures are not recommended, although research is limited in this area for the horse. Lower temperatures (≤5°C) result in reduced developmental potential after storage of bovine ovaries or oocytes when compared with ≥25°C.[33,34] Although we have occasionally received ovaries shipped at approximately 5°C and produced early pregnancies, no foals have resulted. General recommendations are that ovaries collected in close proximity (ideally <1 hour) to the laboratory are maintained at

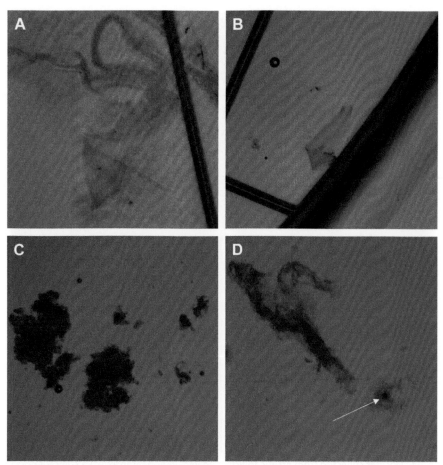

Fig. 13. Examples of granulosa cells from follicles that are mature (*A*), immature (*B*), atretic (*C*), and atretic with an associated oocyte (*D, arrow*).

approximately body temperature (37–38°C), whereas ovaries shipped for longer distances are held at a cool room temperature, within a range of 15 to 24°C, depending on the duration of shipment. The shipping container or method needs to be adequate to prevent high and low temperature fluctuations. Although clinical offspring have been produced from harvested ovaries that were transported for various lengths of time and under different conditions,[27,28,31] the harvesting of oocytes from excised ovaries at the facility of origin and shipment of oocytes instead of ovaries could have a positive impact on results.

OOCYTE SHIPMENTS

Oocytes also can be collected from live mares at one facility and shipped to another facility for ICSI. The shipment of oocytes has gained popularity in the equine industry, as it provides a method to remotely access the expertise and expensive equipment associated with ICSI. Most shipped oocytes are recovered from small, immature follicles. These oocytes can be transported overnight and placed into maturation

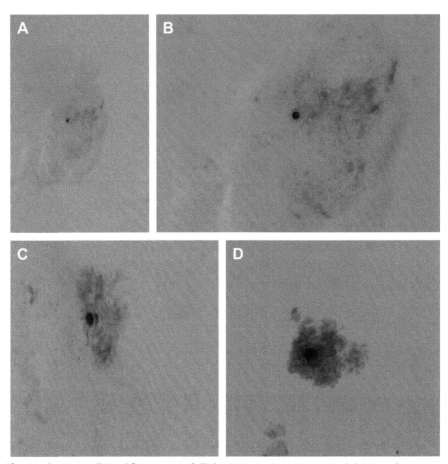

Fig. 14. Oocytes collected from atretic follicles can vary in appearance: (*A*) a cumulus oocyte complex with expansion and some clumping of cumulus cells; (*B*) at higher magnification an oocyte with dark ooplasm is imaged; (*C*) moderate expansion of cumulus cells and a shrunken, fragmented oocyte; and (*D*) dark cumulus cells with some expansion and a tight corona radiata.

medium the following morning, with ICSI performed the next day. Shipment of oocytes from immature follicles versus maturing follicles has the advantage of providing more oocytes, less rigid temperature requirements, and more time flexibility. Oocyte shipments need to be synchronized with the receiving facility, and this should be done before collections. Conditions for shipping immature oocytes originated from methods to hold oocytes without meiotic progression. A medium specifically designated for equine holding (EH) (40% M199 with Earle salts, 40% M199 with Hank salts and 20% fetal bovine serum) was used to hold immature oocytes at room temperature for 18 h without an apparent loss in developmental competence.[1,35] However, when immature oocytes were held at 23°C for 15 hours before being placed in maturation medium, blastocyst development was similar in EH, room-buffered TCM199 (TCM199 with Hank salts and additions of 20% newborn calf serum, 25 μg/mL genta-micin, and 0.3 mmol/L sodium pyruvate) and a commercial embryo-holding medium (EmCare Holding Solution, ICPbio Reproduction, Spring Valley, WI).[3] Oocytes have also been kept in a HEPES-buffered synthetic oviductal fluid for 18 hours with only a marginal decline in developmental competence.[6] In the study, the chromatin configuration of oocytes after holding progressed toward meiotic resumption, suggesting a selection of the most competent oocytes during the holding process.[6]

At this time, most practitioners are shipping oocytes to participating facilities in commercial embryo-holding media, such as SYNGRO (Vetoquinol USA, Inc, Fort Worth, TX) or EMCARE (ICPbio Reproduction, Spring Valley, WI) (EM Carnevale, Colorado State University, Fort Collins, CO; R Foss, Equine Medical Services, Inc, MO; K Hinrichs, Texas A&M University, College Station, TX, personal communication, 2016). Embryo-holding media are buffered for room atmosphere and commercially available, providing a convenient alternative for the practitioner. However, media such as EH (Texas A&M) and TCM199 + Hank salts (Colorado State University) are also being used for in-house holding of oocytes.

For holding and shipping oocytes, nontoxic containers with secure closures should be used. Oocytes have been held and shipped in 1-mL borosilicate glass vials (Shell vials, VWR shell vials; VWR International, Radnor, PA),[25] 5-mL polypropylene culture tubes (Fisher Scientific, Pittsburgh, PA),[3] or cryogenic vials (Nalgene; Fisher Scientific). When packaging containers, a minimal amount of air should remain in the tube, and the cap should be fastened and secured with a layer of Parafilm. Small vials can be placed in larger tubes if needed to properly house them in the shipping container (**Fig. 15**). The optimal temperature for holding immature equine oocytes has not been critically evaluated. Most research has been conducted at "room temperature," leaving some variability, although blastocyst development has been obtained after temperatures of $23^\circ C$[3] and 22 to $25^\circ C$.[6] When temperature-controlled incubators are used, most clinical oocytes are being shipped at $22^\circ C$ (R Foss and K Hinrichs, personal communication, 2016).

Shipment of maturing oocytes can be complicated by timing and incubation conditions. The oocytes need to arrive at an ICSI facility within the interval for normal maturation. This is usually determined based on time from administration of induction drugs to the donor mare, with 36 to 40 hours considered the probable time to ovulation, and

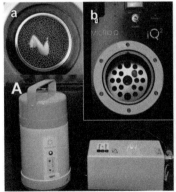
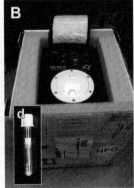
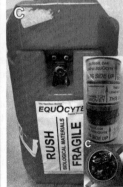

Fig. 15. Containers for shipping equine oocytes include the Minitube incubator (*A*) with a set temperature, rechargeable battery pack, and metal beads within the chamber (a); MicroQ (*B*) with a rechargeable battery, adjustable temperature, and metal tube holder (b); EquOcyte (*C*) with ballast cans and bags in a thermoinsulated container (c) designed to maintain approximate room temperature (c). Oocytes can be packaged in a tube or a tube within a tube (d) to fit within the containers.

the oocyte remaining viable for at least 6 hours after anticipated ovulation. In our laboratory, we usually perform ICSI at 40 to 44 hours after administration of induction compounds to the oocyte donor. This timing is in line with other laboratories, which have performed ICSI at 42 hours[3] or a range of 41 to 46 hours[7] after administration of deslorelin acetate to donors. Long delays in transport will result in the oocyte becoming "aged" and losing viability. In our laboratory, we often organize shipments of maturing oocytes in the following way. Administration of the induction compounds occurs in the evening of the day before oocyte collection. The oocyte is collected in the afternoon of the following day and packaged in transport medium. Gassed culture medium or a medium buffered for room atmosphere (M199 with Hank salts and 25 mM HEPES with the addition of 10% fetal calf serum) has been used for shipping maturing oocytes. The base medium is commercially available and can be made at the shipping facility, or the complete medium usually can be provided from the facility that will be receiving the oocyte. Only one controlled study has been performed to directly compare potential shipping conditions for maturing oocytes.[3] Control oocytes were cultured in medium (45% M199 with Earle salts, 45% Dulbecco modified Eagle medium/F12 with 15 mmol/L HEPES, 10% newborn calf serum, 0.15 mmol/L sodium pyruvate and 25 μg/mL gentamicin) at 37°C and in an atmosphere of 5% O_2, 5% CO_2, and 90% N_2. Blastocyst development rates were high for control oocytes and for oocytes placed in the same gassed medium in a tightly sealed polypropylene culture tube. The use of media buffered for room atmosphere (M199 with Hank salts, 20% newborn calf serum, 25 μg/mL gentamicin, and 0.3 mmol/L sodium pyruvate) resulted in a slightly lower, but not significantly different, blastocyst development rate.[3] Because of the difficulties in gassing transport medium, most clinicians are currently shipping the preovulatory oocytes in M199 with Hank salts, which does not require gas equilibration (EM Carnevale, R Foss, K Hinrichs, personal communication, 2016). Because maturing oocytes are sensitive to temperature changes, they should be shipped at approximately body temperature (37.8–38.2°C). The oocytes will continue the maturation process during transport, and ICSI will be performed the following morning. Shipping via ground services is less expensive and can be more reliable, with the package marked for early arrival. Shipments via air are also acceptable, but the shipper needs to be aware of designated shipper status and package requirements. Connecting flights also can cause delays.

Portable incubators are available for shipping maturing or immature oocytes (see **Fig. 15**). The Minitube incubator (Minitube International, Tiefenbach, Germany) has a battery pack and a container filled with beads to maintain a constant temperature. The beads allow placement of different sizes of tubes, although it is best to place small tubes within a larger tube and plastic covering, as the contents can be jostled during transport. These incubators are preset at a specific temperature by the manufacturer. A second portable incubator has heating and cooling capacities and can be used at variable temperature settings in a wide range that includes room and body temperature (Micro Q; Micro Q Technologies LLC, Scottsdale, AZ), allowing it to be adjusted for the shipment of maturing or immature oocytes and for ICSI-produced embryos. The container includes a metal insert for tubes of different sizes. Immature oocytes also can be shipped in an insulated container with a series of ballast cans (EquOcyte; Hamilton Biovet, Ipswich, MA); the container is marketed as maintaining a temperature within a degree of 22.5°C if used as instructed. In general, the incubators with batteries are set within the range of 37 to 38.2°C for the shipment of maturing oocytes. Immature oocytes are shipped at approximately 22°C. The immature oocytes should not be shipped at body temperature unless appropriate hormones are added to initiate maturation, and the receiving facility can perform ICSI in a timely fashion.

SUMMARY

The development of procedures to collect and mature equine oocytes has resulted in the expansion of assisted reproductive techniques within the equine industry, and the use of ICSI is well-established as a method of assisted fertilization. Oocytes can be collected from maturing or immature follicles from live mares or harvested ovaries. These oocytes can be shipped under defined conditions to a central facility for ICSI. To obtain success with these procedures, the clinician needs to be knowledgeable in the proper methods to collect, identify, and handle oocytes.

ACKNOWLEDGMENTS

Research support provided by The Cecil and Irene Hylton Foundation, and images obtained through the Assisted Reproduction Program at Colorado State University's Equine Reproduction Laboratory, Fort Collins, CO.

REFERENCES

1. Hinrichs K. Application of assisted reproductive technologies (ART) to clinical practice. Am Assoc Equine Pract 2010;56:195–206.
2. Carnevale EM, Coutinho da Silva MA, Panzani D, et al. Factors affecting the success of oocyte transfer in a clinical program for subfertile mares. Theriogenology 2005;64:519–27.
3. Foss R, Ortis H, Hinrichs K. Effect of potential oocyte transport protocols on blastocyst rates after intracytoplasmic sperm injection in the horse. Equine Vet J 2013;45:39–43.
4. Altermatt JL, Suh TK, Stokes JE, et al. Effects of age and equine follicle-stimulating hormone (eFSH) on collection and viability of equine oocytes assessed by morphology and developmental competency after intracytoplasmic sperm injection (ICSI). Reprod Fertil Dev 2009;21:615–23.
5. Choi Y-H, Velez IC, Marcias-Garcia B, et al. Effect of clinically related factors on in vitro blastocyst development after equine ICSI. Theriogenology 2016;85:1289–96.
6. Galli C, Duchi R, Colleoni S, et al. Ovum pick up, intracytoplasmic sperm injection and somatic cell nuclear transfer in cattle, buffalo and horses: from the research laboratory to clinical practice. Theriogenology 2014;81:138–51.
7. Jacobson CC, Choi Y-H, Hayden SS, et al. Recovery of mare oocytes on a fixed biweekly schedule, and resulting blastocyst formation after intracytoplasmic sperm injection. Theriogenology 2010;73:1116–26.
8. Hawley LR, Enders AC, Hinrichs K. Comparison of equine and bovine oocyte-cumulus morphology within the ovarian follicle. Biol Reprod 1995;1:243–52.
9. Colleoni S, Barbacini S, Necchi D, et al. Application of ovum pick-up, intracytoplasmic sperm injection and embryo culture in equine practice. Proc Am Assoc Equine Pract 2007;53:554–9.
10. Bøgh IB, Brink P, Jensen HE, et al. Ovarian function and morphology in the mare after multiple follicle punctures. Equine Vet J 2003;35:575–9.
11. Carnevale EM. Clinical considerations regarding assisted reproductive procedures in horses. J Equine Vet Sci 2008;28:686–90.
12. Vanderwall DK, Woods GL. Severe internal hemorrhage resulting from transvaginal ultrasound-guided follicle aspiration in a mare. J Equine Vet Sci 2002;22:84–6.

13. Velez IC, Arnold C, Jacobson CC, et al. Effects of repeated transvaginal aspiration of immature follicle on mare health and ovarian status. Equine Vet J 2012;44: 78–83.
14. McKinnon AO, Carnevale EM, Squires EL, et al. Heterogenous and xenogenous fertilization of in vivo matured equine oocytes. J Equine Vet Sci 1988;8:143–7.
15. Carnevale EM, Squires EL, Maclellan LJ, et al. Use of oocyte transfer in a commercial breeding program for mares with various abnormalities. J Am Vet Med Assoc 2001;218:87–91.
16. Mari G, Merlo B, Iacono E, et al. Fertility in the mare after repeated transvaginal ultrasound-guided follicular aspirations. Anim Reprod Sci 2005;88:299–308.
17. Vanderwall DK, Hyde KJ, Woods GL. Effect of repeated transvaginal ultrasound-guided follicle aspiration on fertility in mares. J Am Vet Med Assoc 2006;228: 248–50.
18. Hinrichs K, Schmidt AL, Friedman PP, et al. In vitro maturation of horse oocytes: Characterization of chromatin configuration using fluorescence microscopy. Biol Reprod 1993;48:363–70.
19. Alm H, Torner H, Kanitz W, et al. Comparison of different methods for the recovery of horse oocytes. Equine Vet J Suppl 1997;29:47–50.
20. Dell'Aquila ME, Masterson M, Maritato F, et al. Influence of oocyte collection technique on initial chromatin configuration, meiotic competence, and male pronucleus formation after intracytoplasmic sperm injection (ICSI) of equine oocytes. Mol Reprod Dev 2001;60:79–88.
21. Carnevale EM, Ginther OJ. Defective oocytes as a cause of subfertility in old mares. Biol Reprod Mono 1995;1:209–14.
22. Maclellan LJ, Carnevale EM, Coutinho da Silva MA, et al. Pregnancies from vitrified equine oocytes collected from super-stimulated and non-stimulated mares. Theriogenology 2002;58:911–9.
23. Galli C, Colleoni S, Duchi R, et al. Developmental competence of equine oocytes and embryos obtained by in vitro procedures ranging from in vitro maturation and ICSI to embryo culture, cryopreservation and somatic cell nuclear transfer. Anim Reprod Sci 2007;98:39–55.
24. Carnevale EM, Frank-Guest BL, Stokes JE. Effect of equine oocyte donor age on success of oocyte transfer and intracytoplasmic sperm injection. Anim Reprod Sci 2010;121S:S258–9.
25. Hinrichs K. In vitro production of equine embryos: state of the art. Reprod Domest Anim 2010;45(Suppl 2):3–8.
26. Preis KA, Carnevale EM, Coutinho da Silva MA, et al. In vitro maturation and transfer of equine oocytes after transport of ovaries at 12 or 22°C. Theriogenology 2004;61:1215–23.
27. Carnevale EM, Maclellan LJ, Coutinho da Silva MA, et al. Pregnancies attained after collection and transfer of oocytes from ovaries of five euthanatized mares. J Am Vet Med Assoc 2003;222:60–2.
28. Carnevale EM, Maclellan LJ. Collection, evaluation and use of oocytes in equine assisted reproduction. Vet Clin North Am Equine Pract 2006;22:843–56.
29. Carnevale EM, McKinnon AO, Squires EL, et al. Ultrasonographic characteristics of the preovulatory follicle preceding and during ovulation in mares. J Equine Vet Sci 1988;8:428–31.
30. Pierson RA, Ginther OJ. Ultrasonic evaluation of the preovulatory follicle in the mare. Theriogenology 1985;24:359–68.
31. Hinrichs K, Choi Y-H, Norris JD, et al. Evaluation of foal production following intracytoplasmic sperm injection and blastocyst culture of oocytes from ovaries

collected immediately before euthanasia or after death of mares under field conditions. J Am Vet Med Assoc 2012;241:1070-4.

32. Ribeiro BI, Love LB, Choi YH, et al. Transport of equine ovaries for assisted reproduction. Anim Reprod Sci 2008;108:171-9.

33. Wu B, Tong J, Leibo SP. Effects of cooling germinal vesicle-stage bovine oocytes on meiotic spindle formation following in vitro maturation. Mol Reprod Dev 1999; 54:388-95.

34. Yang NS, Lu KH, Gordon I. In vitro fertilization (IVF) and culture (IVC) of bovine oocytes from stored ovaries. Theriogenology 1990;33:352.

35. Choi YH, Love LB, Varner DD, et al. Holding immature equine oocytes in the absence of meiotic inhibitors: Effect on germinal vesicle chromatin and blastocyst development after intracytoplasmic sperm injection. Theriogenology 2006;66: 955-63.

Intracytoplasmic Sperm Injection, Embryo Culture, and Transfer of In Vitro–Produced Blastocysts

CrossMark

Kindra Rader, BS, Young-Ho Choi, DVM, PhD, Katrin Hinrichs, DVM, PhD*

KEYWORDS

- Oocyte • Maturation • ICSI • Blastocyst • Equine • In vitro embryo production

KEY POINTS

- Documentation and preparation are indispensable in a clinical ICSI program to synchronize the handling of oocytes, sperm, and embryo shipments.
- The basic steps in the performance of in vitro embryo production are oocyte collection, oocyte shipment, culture for oocyte maturation, sperm preparation, ICSI, and embryo culture.
- In vitro embryo production requires knowledge of media components and oocyte and embryo culture requirements, skill in oocyte and embryo handling and sperm preparation, and expertise in micromanipulation.
- In our laboratory, current expected performance is that 66% of immature oocytes mature in culture, 1% are lysed during ICSI, 75% cleave after ICSI; 23% (for oocytes recovered from immature follicles) to 38% (for oocytes recovered from dominant stimulated follicles) of oocytes subjected to ICSI develop to blastocysts; blastocysts are shipped to outside embryo transfer centers and the foaling rate per transferred blastocyst is 52%.

INTRODUCTION

Intracytoplasmic sperm injection (ICSI) is a method for in vitro fertilization in which one sperm is injected into the cytoplasm of a mature oocyte to achieve fertilization. This is currently the only repeatable and effective method for in vitro fertilization in the horse, because efficient methods for standard in vitro fertilization, that is, placing sperm and mature oocytes together in media to allow sperm penetration, have not yet been identified.

The authors declare that they have no conflicts of interest in the presentation of this material.
Department of Veterinary Physiology and Pharmacology, College of Veterinary Medicine & Biomedical Sciences, Texas A&M University, 4466 TAMU, College Station, TX 77843-4466, USA
* Corresponding author.
E-mail address: khinrichs@cvm.tamu.edu

Methods for oocyte recovery, maturation, and shipment are discussed elsewhere in this issue. Briefly, immature oocytes are recovered via transvaginal ultrasound-guided follicle aspiration of subordinate follicles existing on the mares' ovaries at any given time. Alternatively, the maturing oocyte is recovered from the dominant preovulatory follicle after gonadotropin stimulation. Mares are shipped to the ICSI laboratory for oocyte recovery, or recovery is performed at the mare's location by a referring practitioner, with recovered oocytes shipped to the desired ICSI laboratory.

For convenience of subsequent micromanipulation scheduling, immature oocytes are held overnight at room temperature before being placed into maturation culture the following morning. Oocytes from dominant stimulated follicles are cultured immediately upon recovery, until about 40 hours after the donor mare received gonadotropin stimulation. Mature (metaphase II [MII]) oocytes, either from in vitro maturation of immature oocytes or from completion of maturation of an oocyte recovered from the dominant stimulated follicle, are subjected to ICSI. Fertilized oocytes are cultured to the blastocyst stage in vitro, then resulting blastocysts are transferred transcervically to recipient mares.

INDICATIONS AND CONTRAINDICATIONS
Indications

ICSI is an effective means of obtaining foals from mares that do not provide embryos for embryo transfer. This may be caused by chronic endometritis, cervical defects, damage to the reproductive tract from previous foals, repeated incidence of hemorrhagic anovulatory follicles, or possibly oviductal problems that prevent fertilization or descent of the embryo into the uterus. We have also found that older mares that no longer efficiently provide embryos, apparently because of age, may be able to produce embryos after oocyte recovery and ICSI.

Indications for ICSI in stallions include old age, in which stallions may no longer produce quantity or quality of semen needed for standard insemination, or death of the stallion or other situations where frozen semen stores are the only existing source of semen. ICSI is useful in these cases because it is conducted with a small number of sperm. In the United States, semen is conventionally frozen in 0.5-mL straws at 200 million sperm per mL, resulting in 100 million sperm per 0.5-mL straw. Frozen semen straws may be cut so that 6 to 10 "ICSI-cuts" are produced; these can be thawed separately, one for each ICSI procedure. Even further, depending on the post-thaw motility of a frozen ejaculate, straws of frozen semen may be thawed, diluted to about 1 million sperm/mL, and refrozen,[1] resulting in hundreds of ICSI doses, each of which may be thawed separately to perform an ICSI procedure, or even themselves cut to allow several ICSI procedures per straw (**Fig. 1**). In this way, the potential of a limited store of frozen semen to produce foals is logarithmically increased.

Contraindications

The success of ICSI is highly variable. In our program, 36% of immature follicle aspirations yield no embryo. However, in other cases, aspiration and ICSI result in production of multiple embryos, so the average embryo production may approach or even exceed one blastocyst per aspiration.

The oocyte recovery procedure, although it has a low rate of complications, is not a completely benign procedure. During transvaginal aspiration (TVA) a needle is passed through the vaginal wall into the peritoneum and ovary, multiple times per ovary in the case of immature follicle aspiration. Potential health risks of transvaginal aspiration

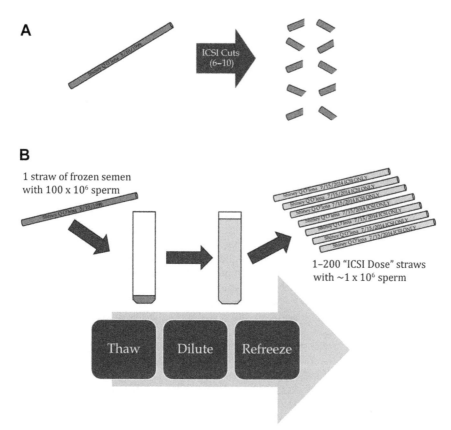

Fig. 1. Methods for increasing the number of ICSI procedures possible with one straw of frozen semen. (*A*) A single standard straw of frozen semen can be sectioned into multiple "ICSI-cuts" or (*B*) may be thawed, diluted, and refrozen into hundreds of "ICSI doses." Depending on the numbers of motile sperm in the ICSI doses, these may also be sectioned into cuts for multiple ICSI procedures.

include rectal tears, bleeding from laceration of major vessels, ovarian infection, abscess or hematoma, and peritonitis.[2,3]

The rate of pregnancy loss after transfer of ICSI-produced embryos (20% or more[4]) is higher than that for transfer of normally-conceived embryos. In addition, although neither our center nor those with which we have contact have had reports of neonatal problems in foals produced by ICSI, the normality of ICSI-produced foals has not been documented.

Because of these drawbacks, ICSI is not a recommended means of obtaining more foals in a given season from a normally-fertile mare with standard quality semen. ICSI should only be used when indications listed previously are present, or if all other assisted reproduction methods have failed.

Although not directly a contraindication, the owner should be aware that performing ICSI is much more costly than is standard embryo transfer. Typically, in our program, taking into account the pregnancy rate after transfer and the pregnancy loss rate, the aspiration and laboratory costs alone of producing an ICSI embryo that goes on to yield a foal is approximately $5000. This is in addition to costs for performing the transfer of the embryo and costs for purchasing and maintenance of the recipient mare.

PROCEDURE
Documentation and Arrangements

Before planning to perform ICSI on a mare's oocytes, the mare owner should contact the desired ICSI laboratory to determine what is required regarding documentation. At A&M, each mare owner signs a contract that outlines the procedures that will be performed, the potential health hazards to the mare undergoing TVA (if TVA is to be performed at A&M), and the likelihood of obtaining no embryos and/or no foals from the ICSI process. Mare owners are also made aware of the possibility that a parentage mix-up could occur and are advised to have all foals, even those not being registered, parentage-tested at birth.

All mare owners should understand the costs involved with ICSI procedures offered by the laboratory chosen, and make decisions accordingly. It is not uncommon for mares to have multiple owners, such as arrangements between partners for first embryos versus second embryos. In these cases at A&M, both owners must sign a contract and state the financial arrangements at the time the contract is signed, or all charges are levied to the legal mare owner who signs a contract. The A&M contract asks for the desired stallions to be designated. At the time of signing the contract, the mare owner must have a breeding contract with each stallion owner. Texas A&M checks with the stallion owner listed to make sure that a breeding contract for this mare is in place and that the stallion owner understands that this is an ICSI breeding. If fresh-shipped semen is to be used, the collection schedule is verified at that time for scheduling purposes.

Because of the potential asynchrony of in vitro production of embryos after TVA of the donor mare (blastocysts equivalent to Day 6 in vivo embryos can be produced up to 11 days after donor mare aspiration), and the potential for multiple embryos to be generated, it is generally necessary for the donor mare owner to use recipient mares. At A&M, we do not have a recipient herd, thus our mare contract also requires the owner to state the embryo transfer center to which the embryos will be shipped, and the owner must have an agreement in place with that center. We do not accept mares for TVA, or oocytes from referring practitioners, if we do not have a signed ICSI contract in place. We also do not accept the mare for TVA or oocytes for ICSI if there is no breeding contract in place, or if the owner does not have an agreement in place with the chosen embryo transfer center.

The referring veterinarian contacts the ICSI laboratory at minimum 1 day before the scheduled TVA, to alert the laboratory that oocytes from the given mare should be expected. When shipping oocytes to the ICSI laboratory, it is vital that documentation accompany the oocytes at all times. This identifying information should include the registered name of the mare and the mare owner's name, address, and contact information, and confirmation of the desired stallion for ICSI. The number of oocytes contained in the shipment should be stated. Semen shipment orders should ideally be placed before the mare undergoes TVA, because collection and shipping schedules may not always match the timeframe of the laboratory performing ICSI. The semen should arrive in the laboratory no later than the day after the oocytes arrive (in this way, semen is not shipped if oocytes are not recovered from the mare). If frozen semen is to be used, additional straws from the desired stallion should be provided, in case of cracking of a straw during thawing. Substitute stallion options should be considered, especially in the case of fresh-shipped semen, in case of accidents or shipment problems for that stallion on the day that his semen is needed. Awareness of this possibility before the day of ICSI may prevent disruption of ICSI proceedings and inability to perform sperm injection on valuable oocytes because of unforeseen circumstances.

In the laboratory, meticulous labeling of each individual mare's oocytes through the entire maturation, ICSI, and embryo culture process, and each stallion's sperm through sperm preparation, is necessary to protect the identity of the oocytes and embryos from the time they are collected to the time each blastocyst is prepared for transfer. In a busy ICSI laboratory, 10 mare-stallion combinations may be fertilized on a given day.

Handling of Oocytes on Receipt at the Laboratory

When immature oocytes are received at Texas A&M University from referring veterinarians, they have typically been shipped overnight in an embryo-holding medium at room temperature. This low temperature supports the oocytes without stimulating them to start maturation.[5] Dishes containing 150-μL droplets of maturation media (M199 with Earle salts [Invitrogen, Carlsbad, CA] with 25 μg/mL gentamicin [Invitrogen], 10% fetal bovine serum [FBS; Invitrogen], and 5 mU/mL follicle-stimulating hormone [Sioux Biochemicals, Sioux Center, IA]), under light white mineral oil (Sigma-Aldrich, St. Louis, MO; or Sage, In-Vitro Fertilization, Inc., Trumbull, CT), are made the evening that the oocytes are recovered, and placed in an incubator at 38.2°C and 5% CO_2 in air to equilibrate before use (**Fig. 2**). Others have reported higher blastocyst rates using a DMEM/F-12-based medium for oocyte maturation.[6] However, when we evaluated this in our system, we found lower blastocyst rates for oocytes matured in DMEM/F-12 (Sigma-Aldrich) than in M199.

The morning after the oocytes were recovered (typically the morning of receipt from referring practitioners), the oocyte holding vial is checked for mare identity, and an appropriate number of equilibrated maturation dishes, labeled on the underside of the dish (not on the dish lids, because these may move from dish to dish) with the mare's full name, are used. The oocytes are removed from the vial, and are washed by transferring them through two droplets of maturation medium, and then are placed into the final 150-μL maturation droplet (up to 15 oocytes per droplet). The dish is placed back into the incubator, and the oocytes are cultured for approximately 30 hours. Because all oocytes are placed in maturation in the morning, this means that ICSI may be performed in the afternoon of the following day. Not all oocytes mature, because the oocytes are collected at different stages of follicle growth or atresia, which lends to variability in their meiotic competence.

If oocytes from dominant, stimulated, preovulatory follicles are received, they are typically maturing at the time of recovery and continue maturing during shipment, and thus must be shipped at body temperature (37°C–38.2°C). Because these oocytes have a large cumulus and are metabolizing during shipment, we recommend that they be shipped in a container with at least 5 mL of medium to avoid either using up nutrients or concentrating metabolic degradation products. Once at the laboratory, these oocytes are incubated at 38.2°C until approximately 40 hours after the donor mare received the ovulatory stimulus, then are subjected to ICSI. The oocytes may be incubated in their sealed vials of shipping medium (typically M199/Hanks salts and 10% FBS) or may be placed in a dish of M199/Earle salts with 10% FBS in an atmosphere of 5% CO_2 in air.

Preparation of Oocytes for Intracytoplasmic Sperm Injection

After the maturation period, the dish containing the oocytes is removed from the incubator and the oocytes are evaluated using a dissection microscope. Cumulus cells surrounding the oocytes are removed (denuded) so that the oocyte itself is visualized. Denuding is done by pipetting in 0.05% hyaluronidase (Sigma-Aldrich) in CZB-M[7] or M199/Hanks salts with 10% FBS. Mature (MII) oocytes are identified

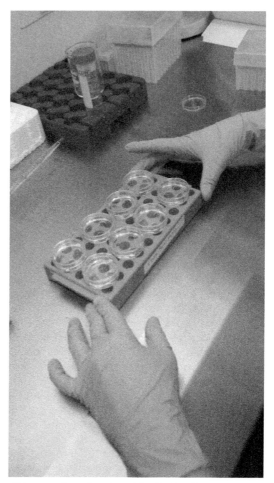

Fig. 2. Maturation dishes ready to be placed in the incubator. Maturation dishes are pre-pared with 150-μL droplets of maturation medium under oil. Use of a plastic tray (in this case a test tube holder) allows multiple dishes to be handled at once for placement into and removal from the incubator.

by presence of the first polar body (**Fig. 3**). After denuding, MII oocytes are placed back into their maturation droplets and returned to the incubator to await ICSI. For oocytes recovered from immature follicles, the maturation rate in our system during the last 3 years has been 66%. For oocytes recovered from dominant stimulated follicles, 91% are in MII and undergo ICSI; the remainder are degenerating and/or broken during denuding.

Preparation of Semen Samples for Intracytoplasmic Sperm Injection

If MII oocytes are available for ICSI, the stallion's semen is prepared. One of the major factors contributing to use of ICSI for foal production is its utility in the case of an aged or deceased stallions, in which there is a limited supply of frozen semen available. Even if a stallion is still actively breeding, use of frozen semen greatly simplifies the arrangements required to have semen in the ICSI laboratory

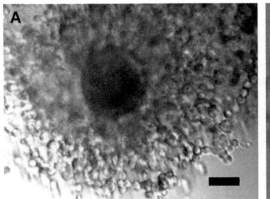
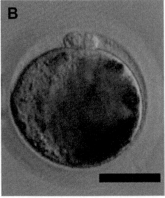

Fig. 3. Morphology of mature equine oocytes before and after denuding of the cumulus. (*A*) Cumulus-intact oocyte. (*B*) Oocyte after denuding of cumulus. The first polar body and an additional bleb of cytoplasm are visible at 12:00 o'clock. Bar = 50 μm.

at the time it is needed. Embryo development after ICSI with fresh or frozen semen is similar.[8] Therefore, frozen semen is one of the most commonly used semen types for ICSI.

If multiple mares are going to the same stallion (this is common if the reason for performing ICSI is limited semen stores and the stallion is breeding only by ICSI), a good management technique is to have these mares undergo TVA on the same day so that their oocytes undergo ICSI on the same day, and one straw or ICSI-cut of semen from that stallion can be used for the oocytes for all the mares going to him on that day.

Cooled semen can also be used for ICSI. Again, only one sperm is needed per oocyte, so breeding farms collecting a stallion for cooled semen for ICSI purposes should be notified of this; they do not have to send a traditional breeding dose and may be able to use it on the farm. Cooled semen can be received the day before ICSI (in which case it is kept in the shipping container overnight, or in the refrigerator in the case of a Styrofoam container), or the morning of the day of ICSI. This latter is dangerous because any delay in delivery of the semen results in oocytes maturing that afternoon not being able to be fertilized.

The most common sperm preparation method used at Texas A&M University is swim-up; this is used when there are adequate sperm numbers. For swim-up, 100 to 200 μL of fresh semen, or frozen-thawed semen (whole original straw, or ICSI-cut of an original straw) is layered under 1 mL of a sperm medium (Sp-CZB[7]) in a 1.5-mL Eppendorf tube, labeled (as are all other tubes used for this stallion) with the stallion's name. After 20-minute incubation at 38.2°C in air, the top approximately 0.6 mL of the medium is collected and placed in a separate Eppendorf tube. This suspension is centrifuged at 327 × g for 3 minutes, the pellet resuspended in 1 mL Sp-CZB, and centrifuged again. The supernatant is removed and the sperm pellet is resuspended in the remaining medium.

If sperm numbers are low (ie, ICSI doses or ICSI-cuts), semen is typically prepared by washing alone. Washing is performed by thawing semen, placing the semen in a 1.5-mL Eppendorf tube, diluting with 1 mL Sp-CZB, and performing centrifugation and resuspension twice as described previously. After the second centrifugation, the supernatant is removed and the sperm is resuspended in the remaining fluid for use for ICSI.

Rarely, because of poor performance of sperm from a specific stallion for ICSI, density gradient separation may be performed. Density gradients are prepared by placing one layer of 3 mL of 40% EquiPure (Nidacon International AB, Mölndal, Sweden) into a 15-mL conical tube. Semen (up to 450 μL) is layered onto the top of the EquiPure and centrifuged at $200 \times g$ for 30 minutes. Following centrifugation, the sperm are washed twice in Sp-CZB and harvested as described previously.

Preparation of Holding Droplets/Dishes for Intracytoplasmic Sperm Injection

ICSI is performed with oocytes and sperm in droplets under oil on the inside of a lid of a 50-mm petri dish. A 50-μL droplet of oocyte holding medium is used to hold the oocytes; we have used CZB-M[7] and M199/Hanks salts with 10% FBS for this purpose. A 3-μL droplet of Sp-CZB containing 7% to 10% polyvinylpyrrolidone (PVP-360, Sigma-Aldrich) is used to hold sperm. Commercial sperm handling and PVP solutions for ICSI are available but we have not yet evaluated their use.

Before the oocytes and sperm are added to the dish, a copy of the original contract is consulted to confirm the identity of the mare and of the stallion undergoing ICSI. The mare and stallion names are written on the bottom of the ICSI dish. The mare name is then checked with the name on the maturation dish from which the oocytes are moved, and the stallion name with the label of the prepared semen tube used to load the sperm droplet.

The ICSI dish with the droplets in place is positioned on the inverted microscope, and 1 μL of final sperm suspension is placed on the surface of the 3-μL PVP medium droplet. The oocyte maturation dish is removed from the incubator and the MII oocytes are placed in the oocyte holding drop. Micromanipulation is performed with the microscope stage heated to 32°C.

Performance of Intracytoplasmic Sperm Injection

At Texas A&M, ICSI is performed under micromanipulation (**Fig. 4**), using one large-diameter (120- to 140-μm outer diameter) holding pipette and one fine (7- to 8-μm outer diameter) injection pipette equipped with a Piezo drill. The oocyte holding

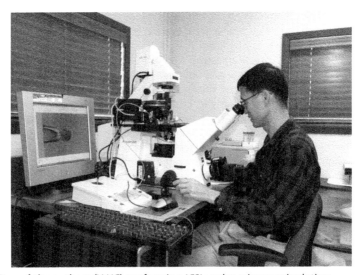

Fig. 4. One of the authors (Y-HC) performing ICSI under micromanipulation.

droplet is evaluated, and using the injection pipette, one oocyte is maneuvered into place at the tip of the holding pipette and secured by aspiration. The PVP-medium droplet is examined and individual motile sperm, with normal morphology, are identified. One sperm is aspirated tail-first into the injection micropipette and when the midpiece enters the pipette, is immobilized using pulses from the Piezo drill. Following immobilization of the sperm, the entire sperm cell is aspirated into the injection pipette, which is then moved to the droplet containing the awaiting oocyte. The oocyte is manipulated with the injection pipette so that the polar body is at 12 or 6 o'clock, and the aspect of the oocyte nearest the holding pipette presents the clearest cytoplasm.

A core of the zona pellucida is bored out with the injection pipette, using Piezo drill pulses, and is discarded (**Fig. 5**). The sperm in the injection pipette is then advanced to the tip of the pipette. The pipette is inserted through the bored hole in the zona, and is advanced into the oocyte to the far side of the oocyte near the holding pipette (**Fig. 6**). The oolemma is broken using a pulse from the Piezo, and the sperm is ejected into the oocyte cytoplasm. This is done without aspirating any of the cytoplasm into the injection pipette.

Embryo Culture

After all oocytes for a given mare have been injected with sperm, the oocytes are placed in a 100-μL droplet of post-ICSI holding medium (CZB-H, or M199/Earle salts

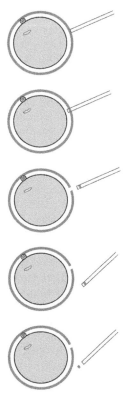

Fig. 5. Boring of the zona with the Piezo drill. The drill allows penetration of the zona and of the oolemma without extensive deformation or manipulation of the oocyte.

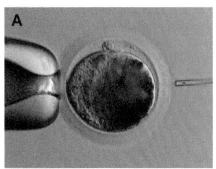
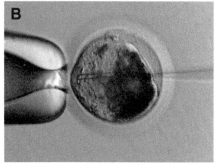

Fig. 6. Sperm injection. (*A*) The oocyte is held by the holding pipette so that the polar body is at 12 or 6 o'clock, and the aspect of the oocyte nearest the holding pipette presents the clearest cytoplasm. (*B*) The injection pipette containing the sperm is inserted through the bored hole in the zona, and is advanced into the oocyte to the far side of the oocyte. The oolemma is broken using a pulse from the Piezo, and the sperm is ejected into the oocyte cytoplasm without aspirating any of the cytoplasm into the injection pipette.

with 10% FBS) and held for approximately 2 hours at 38.2°C in 5% CO_2 in air. The oocytes are checked for lysis; lysed oocytes are discarded and intact oocytes are transferred to embryo culture medium. Few oocytes should undergo lysis; in our system over the last 3 years, loss because of lysis after ICSI has been 1%.

We have used two culture media successfully for equine embryo culture. The simplest system is to use the cell culture medium, DMEM/F-12 (Sigma-Aldrich) with 10% FBS, for the entire culture period.[9] We have also used a human embryo culture medium (Global, Life Global Group LLC, Guilford, CT) for Days 0 to 5 of culture, adding 20 mM glucose to the medium for culture of embryos after Day 5.[10] In either media, embryos are incubated in mixed gas with 5% O_2, 5% to 6% CO_2, and the remainder N_2. The incubator CO_2 setting used should yield a resulting medium pH of about 7.3. The embryos are cultured in microdroplets under oil in groups, with each embryo being allotted 1 μL of medium. No more than five embryos are cultured per droplet.

The embryos are examined for cleavage at Day 5 after ICSI. Any embryo not cleaved is discarded at that time. Embryos that have cleaved are placed into a new droplet of culture medium for development to the blastocyst stage. The cleavage rate for clinical ICSI embryos at Texas A&M over the last 3 years has been 75%.

Embryos are examined daily from Day 7 to Day 10 post-ICSI for blastocyst development. Blastocysts are recognized by formation of an apparent trophoblast layer immediately inside the zona pellucida, with a suggestion of decreased density of the inner aspect of the embryo (**Fig. 7**). Morphologic evaluation of horse blastocysts is challenging, and inexperienced operators are advised to first educate themselves by using practice oocytes for ICSI and embryo culture and then classifying embryos, before staining them with Hoechst to determine their true identity.[11] Over the last 3 years in our clinical ICSI program, the blastocyst rate has been 23% per injected oocyte for oocytes recovered from immature follicles, and 38% per injected oocyte for oocytes recovered from dominant stimulated follicles.

Preparation for Embryo Shipment

It is important to maintain consistent communication with mare owners and embryo transfer practitioners throughout the duration of the embryo culture process to ensure

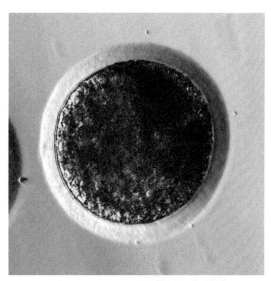

Fig. 7. Equine blastocyst produced by ICSI and in vitro culture. The outer cells, immediately inside the zona pellucida, have formed an apparent trophoblast layer and there is an appearance of decreased density of the inner aspect of the embryo.

availability of recipient mares synchronized to match the needs of in vitro–produced embryos. In vitro–produced blastocysts, no matter what day of culture they are found to have developed, are treated as for Day 6 in vivo embryos. Ideally, the recipient for an in vitro–produced blastocyst should be 4 to 6 days postovulation on the day of transfer. Because blastocysts are available for transfer 7, 8, 9, or 10 days after ICSI, synchronization of recipients is difficult and embryo transfer centers with a large number of recipients to choose from are needed. Communication of the number of oocytes reaching MII gives some idea of the potential need for recipients, and this is narrowed a bit by reporting the number of embryos found to be cleaved at Day 5. This second number can give the maximum blastocysts that might be produced, but cannot predict the actual number; for example, we have had cases where 10 cleaved embryos resulted in one blastocyst, and those where 10 cleaved embryos resulted in seven blastocysts. Ideally, mare owners should be asked to decide, before the day of transfer, the total number of embryos they would like to have transferred, and what additional recipient facilities they would like to use in the case that their first choice of embryo transfer facility does not have availability on the day their embryos are seen to have developed. Embryos not intended for immediate transfer are cryopreserved by slow freezing or vitrification. When blastocysts are identified, the ICSI laboratory confirms recipient mare availability and alerts the embryo transfer center of the impending shipment before scheduling and consigning the packaged embryo.

Packaging Embryos for Fresh Transfer

At A&M, we currently package embryos at room temperature (~22°C) in Bioniche Vigro Embryo Holding Media (Vétoquinol USA Inc, Fort Worth, TX) in a 5-mL polystyrene tube with snap cap (Falcon 352058). The embryo is wrapped in ballast at room temperature and placed in the isothermalizer of an Equitainer (Hamilton Research Inc, Ipswich, MA) with the isothermalizer and coolant cans at room temperature. We ship embryos counter-to-counter same-day air to the embryo transfer centers.

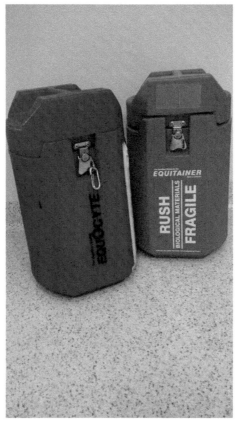

Fig. 8. Containers for shipment of in vitro–produced embryos. Red container: EquOcyte, designed to maintain room temperature. Blue container: Equitainer, designed to cool to ~4°C and maintain that temperature. We use the Equitainer for embryo shipment, but with all materials at room temperature.

Hamilton Research Inc has recently developed another container system, the EquOcyte, designed to maintain oocyte and embryo shipments at room temperature, and we also use this system (**Fig. 8**).

After shipment of embryos to outside embryo transfer centers, the initial pregnancy rate per in vitro–produced blastocyst transferred over the last 3 years in our clinical program has been 72%. However, the embryo loss rate was high (20–27% of established pregnancies) for a pregnancy/foaling rate of 52% per transferred embryo. In 2016, we initiated changes in medium during embryo culture (Global for the first 5 days, followed by DMEM/F-12) which were associated with a reduction in early embryo loss (11% of established pregnancies) but foaling rate is not yet available.

SUMMARY

Documentation and preparation are indispensable in a clinical ICSI program to synchronize the handling of oocytes, sperm, and embryo shipments. The basic steps in the performance of in vitro embryo production are oocyte collection, oocyte shipment, culture for oocyte maturation, sperm preparation, ICSI, and embryo culture. In vitro embryo production requires a knowledge of media components and oocyte and embryo culture requirements, skill in oocyte and embryo handling and sperm preparation, and expertise in micromanipulation. Identification of equine in vitro–produced blastocysts should be verified by staining of practice embryos with Hoechst to verify their stage of development. In our laboratory, expected performance is that 66% of immature oocytes mature in culture, 1% are lysed during ICSI, and 75% cleave after ICSI. Blastocyst development per oocyte subjected to ICSI is 23% for oocytes recovered from immature follicles, and 38% for oocytes recovered from dominant stimulated follicles. After shipment of blastocysts to outside embryo transfer centers, the foaling rate per transferred blastocyst is currently 52%.

REFERENCES

1. Choi YH, Love CC, Varner DD, et al. Equine blastocyst development after intracytoplasmic injection of sperm subjected to two freeze-thaw cycles. Theriogenology 2006;65(4):808–19.
2. Velez IC, Arnold C, Jacobson CC, et al. Effects of repeated transvaginal aspiration of immature follicles on mare health and ovarian status. Equine Vet J Suppl 2012;44(Suppl 43):78–83.
3. Vanderwall DK, Woods GL. Severe internal hemorrhage resulting from transvaginal ultrasound-guided follicle aspiration in a mare. J Equine Vet Sci 2002;22:84–6.
4. Hinrichs K, Choi YH, Love CC, et al. Use of intracytoplasmic sperm injection and in vitro culture to the blastocyst stage in a commercial equine assisted reproduction program. J Equine Vet Sci 2014;34:176.
5. Choi YH, Love LB, Varner DD, et al. Holding immature equine oocytes in the absence of meiotic inhibitors: effect on germinal vesicle chromatin and blastocyst development after intracytoplasmic sperm injection. Theriogenology 2006;66: 955–63.
6. Galli C, Colleoni S, Duchi R, et al. Developmental competence of equine oocytes and embryos obtained by in vitro procedures ranging from in vitro maturation and ICSI to embryo culture, cryopreservation and somatic cell nuclear transfer. Anim Reprod Sci 2007;98:39–55.
7. Choi YH, Chung YG, Walker SC, et al. In vitro development of equine nuclear transfer embryos: effects of oocyte maturation media and amino acid composition during embryo culture. Zygote 2003;11:77–86.
8. Choi YH, Love CC, Love LB, et al. Developmental competence in vivo and in vitro of in vitro-matured equine oocytes fertilized by intracytoplasmic sperm injection with fresh or frozen-thawed sperm. Reproduction 2002;123:455–65.
9. Hinrichs K, Choi YH, Love LB, et al. Chromatin configuration within the germinal vesicle of horse oocytes: changes post mortem and relationship to meiotic and developmental competence. Biol Reprod 2005;72:1142–50.
10. Choi YH, Ross P, Velez IC, et al. Cell lineage allocation in equine blastocysts produced in vitro under varying glucose concentrations. Reproduction 2015;150(1): 31–41.
11. Lewis N, Hinrichs K, Schnaufer M, et al. Effect of oocyte source and transport time on rates of equine oocyte maturation and cleavage after fertilization by ICSI, with a note on the validation of equine embryo morphological classification. Clinical Theriogenology 2016;8:25–39.

Breakthroughs in Equine Embryo Cryopreservation

Edward L. Squires, MS, PhD

KEYWORDS

- Equine • Embryo • Slow cool • Vitrification

KEY POINTS

- Viability of cryopreserved equine embryos less than 300 μm is quite good with either a slow cool method or vitrification.
- Data from commercial embryo transfer stations reported a 50% to 60% pregnancy rate with frozen/thawed equine embryos using vitrification kits.
- Deflating the equine blastocyst of blastocoel fluid before vitrification improved the pregnancy rates of embryos greater than 300 μm.

INTRODUCTION

Embryo recovery and transfer (ET) is a very common technique used in the equine industry that can readily be performed by the veterinarian. This procedure was developed in the late 1970s initially as a treatment for obtaining pregnancies from subfertile mares. Although ET is still used as a treatment of subfertility it is also used to obtain pregnancies from mares that are competing in shows or races. Breeders have also requested this technique as a means of obtaining multiple foals from a mare in a given breeding season. Mares foaling late in the breeding season are often used as embryo donors instead of as broodmares carrying their own foal. This practice allows the foaling mare to remain open so that she can be bred early the following breeding season. One of the advantages of ET that is not realized by the horse industry nearly as much as the cattle industry is cryopreservation of the embryo. This article addresses the barriers to cryopreservation of the equine embryo, provides the state of the art with this technology, and provides insight into breakthroughs that have recently occurred in the technology of cryopreservation of equine embryos.

The author has nothing to disclose.
Department of Veterinary Science, Maxwell H. Gluck Equine Research Center, University of Kentucky, 1500 South limestone Ave, Lexington, KY 40546, USA
E-mail address: edward.squires@uky.edu

Vet Clin Equine 32 (2016) 415–424
http://dx.doi.org/10.1016/j.cveq.2016.07.009
0749-0739/16/© 2016 Elsevier Inc. All rights reserved.

CHANGES IN THE HORSE INDUSTRY IN REGARD TO EQUINE EMBRYO RECOVERY AND TRANSFER

Commercial equine embryo transfer was established in the early 1980s. Because most of the breed registries allowed the use of this technique only from older mares with poor reproductive histories, the embryo recovery per cycle was quite low (30%–50%).[1] Also because there was no protocol for superovulating mares, embryo recovery was based on only one ovulation per cycle. At the very beginning, embryos were transferred by surgical flank incision as soon after collection as possible. To make it even more complicated neither cooled nor frozen semen was generally available; thus, the donor, stallion, and recipient had to be in the same facility. Fortunately, over the next several years several important changes occurred that stimulated the use of embryo transfer:

1. Development of procedures for cooling and shipment of equine semen[1]
2. Change in breed registry regulations allowing the use of ET for any aged mare
3. Procedures for cooling and shipment of equine embryos[2]
4. Offering of continuing education classes for training veterinarians and technicians in the art and science of equine ET
5. The acceptance of ET by the breeder as a means of producing superior genetics
6. Unlimited registration of foals in a given year by most of the major breeds in the United States

With the advent of both cooled and shipped equine semen and embryos, great flexibility in the embryo transfer process was introduced. The donor mare can now be bred with either cooled or frozen semen from any stallion in the country or world (with frozen semen), and the embryo recovered from the mare can be transferred into a recipient on the farm or the embryo shipped to one of the many large recipient stations that have evolved. However, even today most of the equine embryos are transferred fresh (within a few hours of collection or as cooled embryos within 24 hours of collection).

The number of embryo collections and transfers has increased dramatically in the United States, Brazil, and Argentina.[3] Nearly all breeds in the United States use the technique of ET, with the American quarter horse being the leader in ET because this breed produces 60% of all registered foals each year. The primary driver for ET in Argentina would be the polo horse and in Brazil the sport horses and the native breed, mangalarga.

However, the number of embryos frozen has not increased proportionately. A significant difference between embryo transfer in cattle and horses is that a very predictable superovulation regime is available for cattle and typically 6 transferable embryos are available from each flush. In contrast, superovulation is not currently available in horses; consequently, embryo recovery is based on only one ovulation and generally ranges from 50% to 70% embryo recovery per cycle.[1] As a consequence, implementation of cryopreservation procedures in clinical practice has been limited by the number of embryos available and, to a lesser extent, relatively low demand by the equine industry.

Despite the relative limited use of cryopreservation in the horse, there are some distinct advantages:

1. Minimizes the number of recipients and, thus, decreases the cost of embryo transfer
2. Ability to bank embryos, especially from young mares while their performance and the genetic value is being determined

3. Exportation or importation of embryos
4. Less health risks in transporting frozen embryos than importing live animals
5. Collection and cryopreservation of embryos in the off-season so they can be transferred early the following breeding season
6. Cryopreservation of an embryo while genetic testing or sexing is being conducted
7. Ability of in vitro produced embryos to be taken out of culture as a morulae or early blastocyst and frozen at the appropriate size and stage of development

CURRENT TECHNIQUES USED FOR FREEZING EQUINE EMBRYOS

Pregnancy rates with frozen/thawed small equine embryos using the best procedures available have been reported to be similar to cattle embryos and in the range of 50% to 70% per embryo transferred.[1,4–6] When the embryo enters the uterus from the oviduct it is 150 to 220 μm in size and has the morphology of a morula or early blastocyst. Within 0.5 to 1.0 days the embryo will increase in diameter to greater than 300 μm and become a blastocyst. The main factor affecting pregnancy rates of frozen/thawed embryos is the size of the equine embryo.[4,7] Generally the embryo is measured at its greatest width (**Fig. 1**), and those less than 300 μm have good survival and those more than 300 μm have very poor survival (<30% pregnancy rate[7]). This survival rate has been attributed to the structure of the embryo. As an embryo expands beyond 300 μm, the blastocoel fluid increases dramatically and the zona pellucida surrounding the embryo becomes thinner and is replaced by an acellular capsule (**Fig. 2**).[8] It is thought that the large volume of the embryo and the capsule make it difficult for cryoprotectants to penetrate the inner cell mass in sufficient quantity to prevent chilling injury during cryopreservation. Embryos less than 300 μm have the advantage of having a zona pellucida (**Fig. 3**) and no capsule and a relatively small quantity of blastocoel fluid. Thus, the reasons proposed as to why embryos greater than 300 μm do not survive freezing and thawing are as follows:

1. The capsule impedes the penetration of the cryoprotectant.
2. It has been shown that the thickness of the capsule is correlated to the freezability of the embryo.
3. There is a small surface-area-volume ratio.
4. There is a large amount of blastocoel fluid.

It would seem that the solution to the problem would be to only recover embryos less than 300 μm. This recovery has proven to be somewhat difficult, requiring

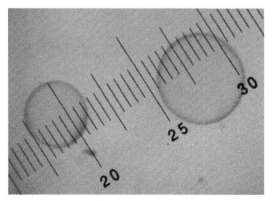

Fig. 1. Measuring an embryo in the dish with an eyepiece micrometer.

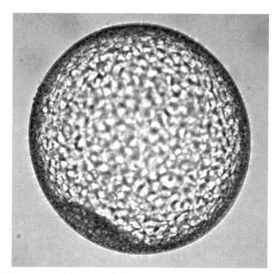

Fig. 2. Expanded blastocyst with an acellular capsule and no zona pellucida.

extensive mare management during the breeding process. Because the equine embryo enters the uterus between 5.5 and 6.0 days[9] and then grows very rapidly in the uterus, the exact time of ovulation is needed. Knowing the exact time of ovulations allows the veterinarian to schedule the flush at the appropriate time to recovery an embryo less than 300 μm. This generally requires performing ultrasound on the mare several times per day while in estrus to pinpoint the time of ovulation. Another approach is to schedule the embryo recovery 8 days after an injection of human chorionic gonadotropin. This approach was shown to provide a high percentage of embryos that were less than 300 μm.[10]

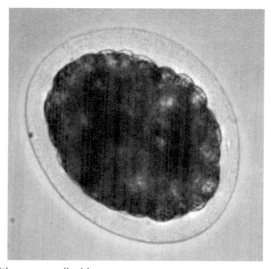

Fig. 3. Embryo with a zona pellucida.

There are 2 ways currently used to freeze equine embryos: slow cool and vitrification. The slow cool method was the initial approach used to freeze equine embryos mainly because the procedure is very similar to what was and is being used in the bovine industry. Pregnancy rates in the range of 60% to 80% have been reported when using this procedure with embryos less than 300 μm. Japanese workers were the first to report the birth of a foal from a frozen/thawed equine embryo in 1982 and in the United States in 1984. Slade and colleagues[4] used glycerol as the cryoprotectant and packaged embryos in 0.5 mL plastic straws. Embryos were cooled at 4°C/min from room temperature to −6°C, seeded, and then held for 15 minutes before cooling at 0.3°C/min to −30°C and finally −0.1°C/min to −33°C. The embryos were then plunged into liquid nitrogen. Eight of 10 classified as early blastocyst (mean diameter 173 μm) resulted in pregnancies, but only 1 of 7 embryos classified as blastocyst resulted in a pregnancy. Based on a commercial embryo transfer program in Argentina[5] using a similar 2-step addition of glycerol and slow cooling of embryos in 0.5-mL straws, a 56% pregnancy rate was obtained.

Thus, the advantage of the slow cool approach is the acceptable pregnancy rate that can be obtained when freezing small, early blastocyst embryos. The main disadvantages with slow cool are the time it takes to freeze an embryo (approximately 2 hours) and the need for an expensive programmable cell freezer. Although many bovine practitioners doing ET would have the knowledge and equipment, it is unusual for bovine ET practitioners to also perform equine ET.

The other option to slow cooling of embryos is the technique of vitrification. This technique is an ultrarapid cooling method that prevents ice crystals from being formed.[3] This method has the advantage of being fast and does not require elaborate equipment. However, it does involve using high concentrations of cryoprotectants; thus, the embryo can be damaged during the process if the procedure is not done properly. In addition, the size of the embryo also effects the survival of the embryo, with only embryos less than 300 μm providing acceptable pregnancy rates after vitrification. The Japanese reported in 1995[11] the viability of vitrified equine embryos. Their criterion for survival was the re-expansion of embryos after vitrification and thawing. Of the embryos less than 300 μm, 13 of 16 re-expanded in culture but only 2 of 8 embryos greater than 300 μm survived.

There are at least 2 commercial vitrification kits available (Vetoquinol USA, Fort Worth, TX and MOFA, Verona, WI), or the solutions can be easily prepared. The procedure for vitrification published by Eldridge-Panuska and colleagues[10] has been used by many for vitrification and the basic procedure is as follows:

- Embryos are recovered 6.0 to 6.5 days after ovulation and measured. Those less than 300 μm are then vitrified. The vitrification solutions (VS) and diluents are taken from the refrigerator and brought to room temperature.
- Four drops of solutions are prepared: diluent, VS1 (1.4 M glycerol in phosphate buffered solution), VS2 (1.4 M glycerol and 3.6 M ethylene glycol), and VS3 (3.4 M glycerol and 4.6 M ethylene glycol).
- Embryos are taken from the holding medium and placed into VS1 for 5 minutes, then VS2 for 5 minutes, and then VS3 for 1 minute. While in the VS3 solution, the 0.25-mL straw is loaded with the embryo in this order: 90 μL of diluent, air space, 30 μL of VS3 with the embryo, air space, and 90 μL of diluent (**Fig. 4**).
- The straw is then heat-sealed and placed in a goblet and exposed to nitrogen vapor for 1 minute before being plunged into liquid nitrogen (**Fig. 5**).
- Embryos are thawed by holding the straw in air for 10 seconds and then a 20°C water bath for 10 seconds. The contents of the straw are shaken several times to

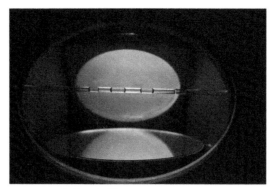

Fig. 4. Embryo in a straw ready for vitrification.

mix the diluent and cryoprotectant and then inseminated in the straw or the contents of the straw are expelled into a dish and then after several minutes of equilibration loaded into a straw and transferred into the mare.

Although this is a fast, simple procedure, there are some potential mistakes that can be made that affect the pregnancy rates of vitrified thawed embryo after transfer:

1. Exposure of the embryo to VS3 solution for greater than 1 minute.
2. Because the embryo may float in the cryoprotectant solution, it may be difficult to find it in the solution. That is why with the VS3 solution, a 30-µL drop is used and the entire drop is aspirated into the straw.

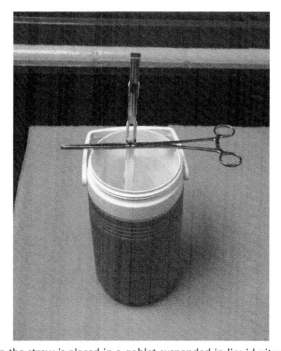

Fig. 5. Embryo in the straw is placed in a goblet suspended in liquid nitrogen.

3. Too much fluid is aspirated when moving the embryo from VS1 to VS2 to VS3, thus, diluting out the levels of cryoprotectants. This dilution can be prevented by using small drops of solutions and pipettes to move the embryo among the drops instead of a 0.25-mL straw.

Eldridge-Panuska and colleagues[10] compared pregnancy rates from vitrification of embryos less than 300 μm and greater than 300 μm. Some were transferred by a direct-straw method and some were taken out of the straw after thawing and reloaded. There was no difference in pregnancy rates with these two methods, and embryos 300 μm resulted in 26 of 48 pregnancies (54%). However, none of the embryos greater than 300 μm survived vitrification and thawing. Another study[6] demonstrated that embryos could be cooled for 16 hours before vitrification and still provide excellent pregnancy rates. They found no difference in pregnancy rates for those transferred immediately after vitrification and those cooled for 16 hours and then vitrified (15 of 20 vs 13 of 20, respectively). This finding means that embryos can be collected on the farm and then cooled and shipped to an embryo transfer facility for subsequent transfer without a decrease in fertility.

Similar to cattle, most of the embryos frozen remain in storage and are not transferred. Therefore, most of the pregnancy data are based on research settings and not commercial data. Recently, however, data were published on pregnancy rates for vitrified/thawed embryos transferred on 2 commercial ET facilities.[12] Most of the embryos were from quarter horse mares flushed 6.0 to 6.5 days after ovulation. Embryos were vitrified with the vitrification kit from Vetoquinol with a slight modification made by each farm. Farm 1 used a pipette instead of a 0.25-mL straw for embryo handling and direct-straw transfer, whereas farm 2 used a 0.25-mL straw for handling but after thawing kept the embryo in holding medium for 1 hour before transfer. Farm 1 reported a 25-day pregnancy rate of 62% based on 421 embryos whereas farm 2 reported a 51% pregnancy rate at 45 days (n = 239). Based on these, it seems that equine embryos can be vitrified and provide good pregnancy rates that are comparable with frozen/thawed bovine embryos.

Unfortunately, acceptable pregnancy rates are still only possible with small morula or early blastocyst embryo whether one is using the slow cool or vitrification procedure. Thus, the challenge is to recover embryos less than 300 μm. Whether one uses slow cool or vitrification is a matter of choice. It does seem as though the room for error is greater for slow cool than for vitrification and that good results can only be obtained with vitrification if one adheres strictly to the published procedures.

MANIPULATING LARGE EQUINE EMBRYOS BEFORE FREEZING

It has been suggested that the reason for the poor freezability of equine blastocyst may be a function of the acellular capsule impeding penetration of cryoprotectants, increased cell numbers, or the large volume of blastocoel fluid. Based on this knowledge, several researchers have tried to modify the large embryo before freezing. Because the thickness of the capsule was shown to be correlated to freezability, one study[7] evaluated whether trypsin could be used to enzymatically thin the capsule and improve embryo survival after freezing/thawing. Embryos greater than 300 μm were assigned to (1) no treatment, (2) trypsin, (3) cytochalasin-B, and (4) combination. Embryos were slow cooled and thawed and transferred. Pregnancy rates were as follows: controls, 4 of 7; cytochalasin-B, 3 of 7; and zero pregnancies for the trypsin and combination group.

Attempts to decrease the amount of blastocoel fluid have been made through galactose dehydration and puncture of the capsule. Barfield and colleagues[13] exposed 46 embryos (300–1350 μm) to 0.6 M galactose for 2 minutes before slow cooling. These investigators stated that there was no advantage to a 2-minute galactose treatment before freezing. They suggested further that a longer dehydration period may be more beneficial because many of the larger embryos showed very little signs of collapse.

The most promising procedure for being able to freeze equine blastocysts is the deflating of the blastocoel cavity before freezing. Most of the studies on deflating equine embryos have dealt with the use of a micromanipulator. Scherzer and colleagues[14] used a laser to create a small opening in the capsule and replaced blastocoel fluid with cryoprotectant before vitrification. Four of 9 blastocysts (>300 μm) resulted in a vesicle on transfer, but only one recipient was still pregnant at day 23. Workers at Texas A&M discovered that equine blastocysts biopsied using a piezo drill collapsed and the blastocoel cavity refilled in 3 hours.[15] In a subsequent study[16] by this same group, embryos that were 300 to 730 μm were biopsied and the blastocoel fluid removed and vitrified. From a series of experiments they determined that embryos up to 650 μm could produce pregnancies after vitrification if greater than 70% of the blastocoel fluid is removed before freezing (near total collapse). Just penetration of the capsule was not sufficient to sustain viability after vitrification. The use of micropipette loader tips for vitrification also seems to be beneficial.

Recently, Diaz and colleagues[17] evaluated several blastocyst micromanipulations and vitrification procedures for day 8 equine embryos. They compared single versus double puncture of the capsule and direct or indirect introduction of cryoprotectants. For the single-puncture technique, the pipette was inserted through one side of the capsule, whereas for the 2-puncture approach, the pipette was inserted completely through the embryo. In both treatments, 95% to 99% of the fluid from the blastocyst was removed. Cryoprotectant was either injected into the embryo or entered passively by exposure. There did not seem to be any benefit to double injection or direct exposure of cryoprotectants. Thus, in a second trial, 6 embryos were punctured once and fluid removed and exposed to cryoprotectants indirectly. Five of 6 vitrified embryos resulted in pregnancies at 25 days. Based on this trial and the studies from Texas A&M, high pregnancy rates can be obtained from large day 7 and 8 equine embryos if most of the blastocoel fluid is removed before vitrification. Unfortunately, these studies were all done using a micromanipulator. These micromanipulators are very expensive pieces of equipment that require skilled technicians to operate. To the author's knowledge there are only 4 commercial companies providing micromanipulation procedures. Most of these facilities have the micromanipulation equipment to be used for in vitro production of embryos. However, it is quite likely that the facilities will provide a service whereby embryos can be shipped to them, deflated, and vitrified. The vitrified embryo could then be shipped back to the owner in a liquid nitrogen container or thawed and transferred to a recipient.

In order to make vitrifying of large equine embryos more economical and practical there needs to be a way of deflating the equine embryo without the use of a micromanipulator. Ferris and colleagues[18] recently reported on a method to manually collapse large equine embryos before vitrification. They compared a manual method against the standard micromanipulator method using a holding pipette and injection pipette. For the manual method, a 25-gauge needle was used to puncture the capsule and remove fluid. All embryos were vitrified in 1.5 M ethylene glycol for 5 minutes then 7 M ethylene glycol and 0.6 M galactose. Once in 7 M solution, they were loaded onto a cryolock device and plunged into liquid nitrogen in 40 seconds. The average size of the embryos was similar in the two groups (687, 663 μm). There was a trend for pregnancy rates at 14 days to be greater for those embryos deflated by the micromanipulator (11 of 15 vs 7 of 15). Pregnancy rates of the embryos collapsed by the micromanipulator were similar to those of fresh transferred embryos (25 of 28). This study confirmed the previous studies demonstrating excellent pregnancy rates with collapsed blastocysts after vitrification and transfer and provided encouragement to further develop a manual means of collapsing large day 7 and 8 embryos.

FUTURE OF EQUINE EMBRYO FREEZING

As the number of equine embryo transfers has increased dramatically for fresh and cooled embryos, the number of embryos frozen has not increased proportionately. In cattle, nearly 60% of the bovine embryos recovered are frozen. This percentage in the horse is estimated to be only 2% to 5% of the embryos collected even though freezing embryos could decrease the cost to maintain recipients and provide increased flexibility. Before an increase in the number of equine embryos frozen increases, several developments will have to occur:

1. Be able to consistently superovulate mares so that extra embryos are available for freezing
2. Either develop a means of hastening the embryo through the oviduct so that small embryos can be obtained consistently or
3. Improve on the system of manually deflating the large embryos before vitrification
4. Develop new international markets for frozen/thawed equine embryos

REFERENCES

1. McCue PM, Squires EL. Equine embryo transfer. Jackson (WY): Teton NewMedia; 2015. p. 84–7.
2. Douglas-Hamilton DH, Osol R, Osol G, et al. A field study of the fertility of transported equine semen. Theriogenology 1984;22:291–304.
3. Stout TA. Cryopreservation of equine embryos: current state-of-the-art. Reprod Domest Anim 2012;47(Suppl 3):84–9.
4. Slade NP, Takeda T, Squires EL, et al. A new procedure for the cryopreservation of equine embryos. Theriogenology 1985;24(1):45–58.
5. Lascombes FA, Pashen RL. Results from embryo freezing and post-ovulation breeding in a commercial embryo transfer programme. Proc 5th International Symposium on Equine Embryo Transfer. Saari (Finland): Havemeyer Foundation Monograph Series 3; 2000. p. 95–6.
6. Hudson JJ, McCue PM, Carnevale EM, et al. The effects of cooling and vitrification of embryos from mares treated with equine follicle-stimulating hormone on pregnancy rates after nonsurgical transfer. J Equine Vet Sci 2006;26(2):51–4.
7. Maclellan LJ, Carnevale EM, Coutinho da Silva MA, et al. Cryopreservation of small and large equine embryos pre-treated with cytochalasin-B and/or trypsin. Theriogenology 2002;58:717–20.
8. Betteridge KJ, Eaglesome MD, Mitchell D, et al. Development of horse embryos up to twenty-two days after ovulation: observations on fresh specimens. J Anat 1982;135:191–209.
9. Battut I, Colchen S, Fieni F, et al. Success rates when attempting to nonsurgically collect equine embryos at 144, 156 or 168 hours after ovulation. Equine Vet J 1997;(25):60–2.
10. Eldridge-Panuska WD, di Brienza VC, Seidel GE, et al. Establishment of pregnancies after serial dilution or direct transfer by vitrified equine embryos. Theriogenology 2005;63(5):1308–19.

11. Hochi S, Fujimoto T, Oguri N. Large equine blastocysts are damaged by vitrification procedures. Reprod Fertil Dev 1995;7(1):113–7.

12. Squires EL, McCue PM. Cryopreservation of equine embryos. J Equine Vet Sci 2016;41:7–12.

13. Barfield JP, McCue PM, Squires EL, et al. Effect of dehydration prior to cryopreservation of large equine embryos. Cryobiology 2009;59(1):36–41.

14. Scherzer J, Davis C, Hurley DJ. Laser-assisted vitrification of large equine embryos. Reprod Domest Anim 2011;46(6):1104–6.

15. Choi YH, Gustafson-Seabury A, Velez IC, et al. Viability of equine embryos after puncture of the capsule and biopsy for preimplantation genetic diagnosis. Reproduction 2010;140(6):893–902.

16. Choi YH, Velez IC, Riera FL, et al. Successful cryopreservation of expanded equine blastocysts. Theriogenology 2011;76(1):143–52.

17. Diaz F, Bondiolli K, Paccamonti D, et al. Cryopreservation of day 8 embryos after blastocyst micromanipulation and vitrification. Theriogenology 2016;85:894–903.

18. Ferris RA, McCue PM, Trundell DA, et al. Vitrification of large equine embryos following manual or micromanipulator-assisted blastocoele collapse. J Equine Vet Sci 2016;41:64.

Hormone Therapy in Clinical Equine Practice

Patrick M. McCue, DVM, PhD

KEYWORDS

- Equine hormone therapy • Equine reproductive management
- Clinical equine practice

KEY POINTS

- The most common hormone therapies in broodmare management are prostaglandins, oxytocin and ovulation induction agents such as human chorionic gonadotropin and deslorelin acetate.
- A practical technique for induction of a timed ovulation for breeding mares with frozen semen is to administer deslorelin at 8:00 pm and anticipate ovulation approximately 40 hours later.
- Evaluation of the ovarian follicle population at the time of prostaglandin administration is helpful in prediction of the interval to subsequent ovulation.
- Administration of altrenogest (0.044 mg/kg, PO, q 24 h) is the most effective and consistent technique for suppression of behavioral estrus.
- Pretreatment of mares with estradiol prior to initiation of dopamine antagonist (ie, domperidone) therapy enhances prolactin secretion for induction of lactation in a nurse mare.

STIMULATION OF FOLLICULAR DEVELOPMENT

Hormone therapy has been used to advance the first ovulation of the year in seasonally anestrous mares, stimulate follicular development in postpartum acyclic mares, and promote development of multiple follicles in cycling mares. The most successful strategies have incorporated natural or recombinant equine follicle-stimulating hormone (FSH) or low doses of a gonadotropin-releasing hormone (GnRH) agonist (**Table 1**).

Administration of purified equine FSH (eFSH) or recombinant equine FSH (reFSH) has been reported to be successful in stimulation of follicular development in seasonally anestrus mares.[1,2] Unfortunately, there are no equine FSH products commercially available currently.

An alternative is twice daily low-dose (10–125 µg) administration of a GnRH agonist such as deslorelin or buserelin.[3] Mares in spring transition (ie, with follicles ≥25 mm in diameter) are more likely to respond than mares in deep winter anestrus (ie, follicles <20 mm in diameter). Mares in deep winter anestrus that do respond to low-dose

Equine Reproduction Laboratory, College of Veterinary Medicine and Biomedical Sciences, Colorado State University, 3101 Rampart Road, Ft. Collins, CO 80523, USA
E-mail address: pmccue@colostate.edu

Vet Clin Equine 32 (2016) 425–434
http://dx.doi.org/10.1016/j.cveq.2016.07.001
0749-0739/16/© 2016 Elsevier Inc. All rights reserved.
vetequine.theclinics.com

Table 1
Hormone therapy to induce follicular development in acyclic mares

Hormone	Dosage, Route, Frequency
Buserelin	10–50 µg, IM, q 6 h to 12 h
Deslorelin	10–50 µg, IM, q 6 h to q 12 h
eFSH	12.5 mg, IM, q 12 h
reFSH	0.65 mg, IM, q 12 h

Abbreviations: eFSH, equine follicle-stimulating hormone; IM, intramuscularly; q, every; reFSH, recombinant equine FSH.

GnRH agonist therapy are more likely to revert back to anestrus after treatment is discontinued than mares initially treated during spring transition. In general, follicular development is evident within 3 to 5 days after the onset of therapy. It is recommended that human chorionic gonadotropin (hCG) be administered to induce ovulation of a follicle stimulated by low-dose GnRH therapy.

Administration of progesterone or progestins during deep seasonal anestrus will not stimulate follicular development.[4,5] However, progesterone treatment near the end of spring transition can be used to synchronize or "program" the day of the first ovulation of the year. Common protocols include administration of 0.044 mg/kg of altrenogest once daily for 14 to 18 days or administration of a combination of progesterone (150 mg) and estradiol (10 mg) once daily for 10 days, with administration of a dose of prostaglandins on the last day of therapy.[6]

INDUCTION OF OVULATION

Induction of ovulation is advantageous if a mare is in a timed breeding, shipped semen, frozen semen, or embryo transfer program. In addition, in mares with a history of accumulating fluid in the uterus following mating or insemination, it may be beneficial to induce ovulation and limit the number of times the mare has to be bred.

hCG was first used for induction of ovulation of mares in 1939. The biological action of hCG is due to its inherent luteinizing hormone (LH)-like activity. hCG is generally administered when a mare is in estrus with a follicle ≥35 mm in diameter and endometrial edema is present (**Table 2**). Ovulation is induced in 85% to 90% of mares within 48 hours, with an average of 36 hours after hCG administration.[7] hCG is most effective in inducing ovulation in young to middle-age mares receiving the hormone for the first 2 or 3 times within a single breeding season. Efficacy at inducing a timed ovulation may be somewhat reduced if hCG is given to a mare repeatedly during the same breeding season.

Table 2
Hormone therapy to induce ovulation in cycling mares

Hormone	Dosage, Route, Frequency
Buserelin	1–1.5 mg, IM, once
Deslorelin	1.8 mg, IM, once
Histrelin	0.5–1.0 mg, IM, once
Human chorionic gonadotropin	1500–2500 units, IV or IM, once

Abbreviations: IM, intramuscularly; IV, intravenous.

Potent agonists of GnRH, such as deslorelin (SucroMate and Ovuplant), buserelin, and histrelin also have been used to induce ovulation in cycling mares[8,9] (see **Table 2**). Administration of a GnRH agonist will stimulate LH release from the anterior pituitary, which will subsequently stimulate follicle maturation, ovulation, and formation of the corpus luteum. GnRH agonist administration will induce ovulation in 90% to 95% of mares within 48 hours, with an average of approximately 40 hours.[10] A convenient strategy to induce a timed ovulation in a mare being inseminated with frozen semen is to administer a GnRH agonist at 8:00 PM and anticipate ovulation at approximately 12:00 noon, 40 hours later (**Box 1, Fig. 1**).

PREGNANCY SUPPORT

Progesterone production by the corpus luteum is required for maintenance of pregnancy during the first 2 to 3 months of gestation. Progesterone levels less than 4.0 ng/mL are associated with an increased risk of pregnancy loss. Administration of exogenous progesterone for "pregnancy support" and the risk of pregnancy loss due to "progesterone deficiency" are controversial topics.[11]

Progesterone/progestin supplementation for mares at risk is usually initiated either 1 to 2 days after ovulation is detected, after ultrasonographic detection of a pregnancy with concurrent presence of uterine edema and/or a small or absent corpus luteum, or measurement of low plasma progesterone levels (**Table 3**). Therapy is often continued until day 120 of pregnancy, at which time production of progesterone by the placenta is adequate to maintain pregnancy.

Supplemental progesterone administration may be used to support problem pregnancies or pregnancies at risk due to placentitis, endotoxemia, colic, or other medical problems. In these instances, altrenogest is commonly given at twice the "normal" dose (ie, 0.088 mg/kg) during the time the mare is at high risk or altrenogest therapy may be continued for the duration of the pregnancy. Additional treatments may include flunixin meglumine, antibiotics, or other drugs, depending on the specific medical condition.

LUTEOLYSIS AND SHORT-CYCLING

Luteolysis or destruction of the corpus luteum is the basis of therapeutic applications, such as short-cycling, estrous synchronization, treatment of a persistent corpus luteum, and termination of pregnancy. The equine corpus luteum takes approximately 5 days to become fully developed or mature and be responsive to prostaglandins. Administration

---

Box 1
Hormone therapy and reproductive management strategy for mares being bred with frozen semen

- Day 1
  - Administer deslorelin at 8:00 PM; anticipate ovulation in 40 hours (12:00 noon).

- Day 2
  - Ultrasound at 8:00 AM, 2:00 PM, and 8:00 PM to monitor follicle status.

- Day 3
  - Ultrasound at 8:00 AM (inseminate if a second dose of frozen semen is available); ultrasound at 12:00 noon to confirm ovulation (inseminate postovulation); if not ovulated, recheck at 8:00 PM, and so on.

- Day 4
  - Ultrasound at 8:00 AM to monitor for uterine fluid accumulation.

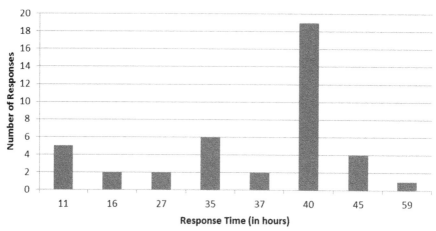

Fig. 1. Interval from deslorelin (SucroMate) administration at 8:00 PM to subsequent ovulation in mares being inseminated with frozen semen postovulation.

of prostaglandins early in the postovulation period will adversely affect development of the corpus luteum. Repeated administration in the postovulatory period will result in failure of the corpus luteum to form (antiluteogenic effect).[12] Estrous synchronization may be achieved by administration of 2 doses of prostaglandins 14 days apart.

Prostaglandin products used in the horse include cloprostenol sodium and dinoprost tromethamine administered as an intramuscular (IM) injection (**Table 4**). Side effects of prostaglandin treatment include mild to moderate sweating, abdominal discomfort, and transient diarrhea.

It is recommended that mares be examined by ultrasound before administration of prostaglandins to confirm that it is the correct mare, a corpus luteum is present, she is not pregnant, and determine the diameter of the largest ovarian follicle. Overall, the average interval to ovulation following prostaglandin administration is 8.4 ± 2.5 days, and is inversely proportional to the diameter of the largest follicle at time of treatment (**Table 5**).[13] Large diestrous follicles (≥35 mm) exhibit 1 of 3 outcomes following prostaglandins treatment: ovulation within 48 hours in the absence of uterine edema (14.5%), ovulation after 48 hours accompanied by uterine edema (75.4%), or regression without ovulation followed by emergence of a new follicular wave (10.1%) (**Fig. 2**).

Elective termination of a pregnancy or a potential pregnancy may be indicated following an unplanned mating of a mare, breeding a mare with the wrong stallion, or other clinical situations. Administration of a single dose of prostaglandins is usually sufficient for complete luteolysis and termination of pregnancy from day 5 postovulation until formation of the secondary corpora lutea. Multiple doses of prostaglandins

Table 3	
Hormone therapy for maintenance of pregnancy	
Hormone	**Dosage, Route, Frequency**
Altrenogest	0.044 mg/kg, orally, q 24 h
Altrenogest (high-risk pregnancy)	0.088 mg/kg, orally, q 24 h or 0.044 mg/kg, orally, q 12 h
Progesterone	200 mg, IM, q 24 h
Progesterone, long acting	1500 mg, IM, q 7 d

Abbreviations: IM, intramuscularly; q, every.

Table 4 Hormone therapy doses for prostaglandins in mares	
Hormone	**Dosage, Route, Frequency**
Cloprostenol	250 µg, IM, once
Dinoprost tromethamine	10 mg, IM, once

Abbreviation: IM, intramuscularly.

may be required for complete luteolysis and termination of a pregnancy after day 35. Treated mares should be reevaluated 5 to 10 days later to confirm that the pregnancy is no longer present.

ECBOLIC DRUGS

Stimulation of uterine contractions is used clinically for evacuation of uterine fluid, induction of labor, and management of retained placentas. The 2 most common hormones with ecbolic effects used in equine practice are oxytocin and prostaglandins (**Table 6**).

Oxytocin administration results in uterine muscular contractions for 30 to 45 minutes. Oxytocin may be administered 1 to 4 or more times per day in an attempt to evacuate fluid from the uterus of older mares or mares with persistent mating–induced endometritis.

Prostaglandin administration stimulates uterine contractions for 2 to 4 hours and may be more effective at evacuation of uterine fluid than oxytocin in some mares.

Administration of prostaglandins to mares either the day ovulation is detected or for 1 to 2 days after ovulation adversely affects the development of the corpus luteum and is associated with a reduction in pregnancy rate. In contrast, prostaglandin treatment before ovulation does not affect corpus luteum function. Oxytocin does not have any adverse effects on corpus luteum development when administered either before or after ovulation. Consequently, prostaglandins or oxytocin may be used to evacuate uterine fluid before ovulation, but oxytocin is a more appropriate choice for treatment after ovulation is detected.

SUPPRESSION OF ESTRUS

Expression of behavioral estrus can have a profound negative effect on training and performance in some mares. Consequently, hormone therapy for suppression of estrus is common in the equine industry. Progesterone is the hormone that naturally suppresses expression of behavioral estrus. Administration of the synthetic progestin

Table 5 Interval from prostaglandin administration in diestrus to subsequent ovulation in mares with a dominant follicle less than 35 mm in diameter		
Follicle Size, mm	**Number of Cycles**	**Interval to Ovulation, d**
<10	6	11.8 ± 1.1^a
10–14	74	10.2 ± 0.2^b
15–19	83	9.1 ± 0.2^c
20–24	118	9.1 ± 0.2^c
25–29	122	8.0 ± 0.2^d
30–34	37	7.8 ± 0.5^d

[a–d] Different superscripts within the column indicate significant differences (p<0.05).

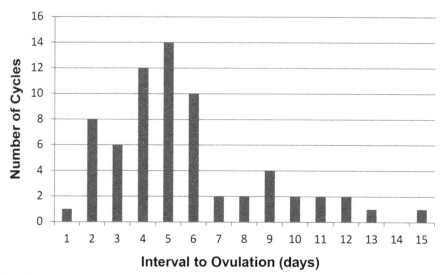

Fig. 2. Interval from prostaglandin administration to subsequent ovulation in mares with a large diestrous follicle (≥35 mm in diameter).

altrenogest once daily is generally effective at suppression of estrus in most mares. Altrenogest treatment should be initiated at least 2 to 3 days before a performance event to allow sufficient time for behavioral modification. It is not recommended to use IM progesterone/progestin products for suppression of estrus in performance mares because of the potential for inflammation at the injection site.

Administration of 60 units of oxytocin IM once or twice daily from day 7 to 14 of the estrous cycle has been reported to result in prolongation of the corpus luteum (pseudopregnancy) in approximately 60% to 70% of mares treated and may be useful as a means of estrous suppression.[14]

Cattle implants containing progesterone and estradiol have been administered to horses in an attempt to suppress heat. However, the implants do not suppress estrus due to the low amount of progesterone in the implants and the designed slow release rate (150 days).[15] Consequently, the use of cattle implants for suppression of estrus in performance mares is not supported or recommended.

Other synthetic progestins, such as medroxyprogesterone acetate, hydroxyprogesterone caproate, norgestomet, and megestrol acetate have also been administered to mares in an attempt to block estrus or maintain pregnancy. Unfortunately, none of the synthetic progestins other than altrenogest are effective in suppression of estrus or maintenance of pregnancy in mares because they do not bind adequately to the equine progesterone receptor. Consequently, although these products may appear to be convenient, they should not be used in horses because of lack of efficacy.

Table 6		
Hormone therapy doses of ecbolic drugs used in equine reproduction		
Hormone	**Dosage, Route, Frequency**	**Indication**
Cloprostenol	250 μg, IM, once	Stimulation of uterine contractions for evacuation of uterine fluid
Oxytocin	20 units, IV or IM, q 6 h to q 24 h or as needed	Stimulation of uterine contractions for evacuation of uterine fluid

Abbreviations: IM, intramuscularly; IV, intravenous; q, every.

Administration of a vaccine against GnRH also has been used for suppression of estrus as well as contraception in mares.[16,17]

Sterilized glass marbles have been inserted into the uterus of mares for the purpose of estrous suppression. Presence of a marble within the uterine lumen may induce formation of a persistent corpus luteum and elevated progesterone levels for 2 to 3 months. However, efficacy at inducing a persistent corpus luteum is low and recent reports have indicated that complications may occur in some mares, such as uterine infections, fracture of the marble, and difficulty in removal of the marble.[18]

STIMULATION OF BEHAVIORAL ESTRUS

Estradiol-17β may be administered to an ovariectomized, seasonally anestrous or acyclic mare to stimulate behavioral estrus and allow the mare to be used as a tease mare or jump mare for semen collection (**Table 7**). Estradiol administration will also result in a profound increase in uterine edema and promote cervical relaxation. Estradiol will not stimulate behavioral estrus when administered to a cycling mare in diestrus when progesterone levels are elevated. Conjugated estrogens (ie, estradiol cypionate or estradiol valerate) will have a longer half-life and similar biological effects as the natural hormone estradiol-17β.

INDUCTION OF LABOR

Oxytocin is the most common hormone used in equine practice to induce labor. Routine induction of labor is not recommended and should be performed only if the *in utero* fetus is sufficiently mature to survive after induced delivery. The following guidelines may be used to determine if the mare qualifies for induction: (1) a gestation length of at least 330 days, (2) significant udder development and engorgement of the teats with colostrum, (3) relaxation of the sacrosciatic ligaments and vulva, (4) elevation in milk calcium, and (5) softening of the cervix as detected during a digital vaginal examination.

A low-dose protocol for induction of labor involves administration of 5.0 IU (0.25 mL of a 20 IU/mL product), intravenously (IV), followed by 10 IU 15 minutes later. The mare will usually rupture her chorioallantoic membrane approximately 10 minutes after the second dose of oxytocin and deliver the fetus within the subsequent 5 to 15 minutes.[19,20]

INDUCTION OF LACTATION

Failure of udder development and lactation may occur in pregnant mares grazing on pastures with tall fescue grass infested with an endophytic fungus. Agalactia also may occur in situations other than fescue toxicosis, such as a young mare giving birth to her first foal. Absence or inadequate lactation may result in failure of passive transfer of antibodies to the newborn foal and inadequate nutrition for a growing foal.

Lactation can be stimulated in mares by administration of a dopamine antagonist, such as domperidone or sulpiride (**Table 8**). Pretreatment with estradiol enhances the effect of dopamine antagonist therapy on stimulation of prolactin secretion.

Table 7	
Hormone therapy using estrogens in equine reproduction	
Medication	**Dosage, Route, Frequency**
Estradiol (E₂)	5–10 mg, IM, every 4–7 d
Estradiol cypionate (ECP)	5–10 mg, IM, every 2–4 wk

Abbreviation: IM, intramuscularly.

Table 8 Hormone therapy to induce lactation in mares		
Hormone	Dosage, Route, Frequency	Indications
Domperidone	1.1 mg/kg, PO, q 24 h	Stimulation of lactation in postpartum mares and induction of lactation in nurse mares
Sulpiride 5% suspension	0.5–1.0 mg/kg, IM, q 12 h to q 24 h	Stimulation of lactation in postpartum mares and induction of lactation in nurse mares

Abbreviations: IM, intramuscularly; PO, oral; q, every.

Dopamine antagonists also have been used to induce lactation in nurse mares to be used for adoption of orphaned foals. The optimal choice for a nurse mare would be a mare that has foaled previously, lactated appropriately, and exhibited good maternal behavior (Box 2).

RETAINED PLACENTA

Retention of the fetal membranes is one of the most common postpartum problems in the mare. An equine placenta is considered to be pathologically retained at 3 hours postpartum. Retention may include the entire chorioallantoic membrane or just the tip of the nonpregnant horn. The incidence of retained placentas increases in mares with dystocia, prolonged gestation, hydrops, cesarean surgeries, or induced labor. Complications associated with retained fetal membranes include metritis, laminitis, septicemia, and death.

Therapy for retained placenta in the horse include administration of oxytocin or prostaglandins, infusion of water in the allantoic cavity (Burns technique), or infusion of water into an umbilical blood vessel.[21] Additional treatments may include uterine lavage, intrauterine antibiotics, parenteral antibiotics, nonsteroidal anti-inflammatory drugs, and tetanus toxoid.

CERVICAL RELAXATION

Insemination of a mare in estrus with a tightly closed cervix will usually result in retention of inflammatory fluid in her uterus, as her normal uterine contractions will be ineffective at evacuation of dead spermatozoa, inflammatory cells, and fluid. Topical application of prostaglandin E_1 (Misoprostol) has been used in an attempt to promote cervical relaxation in mares (ie, older maiden mares). Misoprostol cervical cream is

---

Box 2
Protocol for induction of lactation in a nurse mare

- Select a calm, gentle mare that has given birth and lactated previously.
- Administer estradiol (5 mg) intramuscularly once per day for 2 to 3 days. Potentially continue estradiol therapy every other day during the first few days of dopamine antagonist treatment.
- Begin daily administration of domperidone (1.1 mg/kg, orally, once daily).
- Start hand milking several times daily as the mammary gland increases in size and secretions start to be produced.
- Introduce the foal after the mare has started to produce milk.

available through various veterinary compounding pharmacies. Unfortunately, few published scientific data exist on the effectiveness of misoprostol to induce cervical relaxation in mares. Other options to promote cervical relaxation include administration of estradiol 17β, cloprostenol, N-butylscopolammonium bromide (Buscopan), and manual dilation. Reproductive management of affected mares would include artificial insemination once immediately before or at time of ovulation, uterine lavage 4 to 6 hours after insemination, and administration of oxytocin to promote uterine contractions during the lavage procedure.

MANAGEMENT OF BLOCKED OVIDUCTS

Amorphous globular masses consisting of mucus, collagen, and degenerated cells have been noted to occlude the oviductal lumen of some mares. Oviductal blockage may cause reduced fertility by impeding movement of spermatozoa proximally up the oviduct toward the site of fertilization or block transport of the developing embryo distally down the oviduct toward the uterus.

Diagnosis of oviductal blockage in a mare is difficult. Passage of starch granules or fluorescent microspheres down the oviduct into the uterus and the ability of fluid to pass proximally or distally through a cannulated oviduct have been used in an attempt to diagnose the presence or absence of a blockage.

Laparoscopic application of prostaglandin E_2 gel (Prepidil Gel; dinoprostone cervical gel) to the surface of the oviducts results in dilation of the oviduct and potential resolution of an oviductal blockage.[22] Topical application of prostaglandin E_2 has been reported to increase pregnancy rates in mares with suspected oviductal obstruction. An alternative therapeutic option for blocked oviduct is flushing the oviduct from a ventral midline laparotomy using a retrograde approach or normograde approach. Unfortunately, cannulation of the oviduct through the uterotubular junction using an approach through the uterine lumen is exceedingly difficult.

INCREASING LIBIDO IN STALLIONS

Some stallions may exhibit poor libido in the breeding shed. In many instances this behavior is due to adverse experiences, such as being disciplined for exhibiting sexual interest in mares during performance or training, showing spontaneous erection or masturbation, or being mishandled. Behavioral signs may include failure to show interest in mares, failure to gain an erection, anxiety when around mares, and potentially inappropriate behavior around mares.

Management options include reconditioning training, with controlled exposure to a gentle mare, patience, reinforcement-based handling. Therapeutic options may include administration of anxiolytic medications, such as diazepam (0.05 mg/kg slow IV, 5–7 minutes before breeding) or GnRH, if the poor libido is due to low androgens (50–100 μg, IM, IV, or subcutaneously, 1 to 2 hours before breeding).

REFERENCES

1. Meyers-Brown GA, McCue PM, Troedsson MHT, et al. Induction of ovulation in seasonally anestrous mares under ambient lights using recombinant equine FSH (reFSH). Theriogenology 2013;80:456–62.
2. Niswender KD, McCue PM, Squires EL. Effect of purified equine follicle-stimulating hormone on follicular development and ovulation in transitional mares. J Equine Vet Sci 2004;24:37–9.

3. McCue PM. In: Dascanio J, McCue PM, editors. Management of seasonal anestrous: hormone therapy. In: Equine reproductive procedures manual. Ames (IA): Wiley-Blackwell; 2014. p. 146–8.

4. McCue PM, Logan NL, Magee C. Management of the transition period: hormone therapy. Equine Vet Educ 2007;19:215–21.

5. McCue PM, Patten M, Denniston D, et al. Strategies for using eFSH for superovulating mares. J Equine Vet Sci 2008;28:91–6.

6. Taylor TB, Pemstein R, Loy RG. Control of ovulation in mares in the early breeding season with ovarian steroids and prostaglandin. J Reprod Fertil Suppl 1982;32: 219–24.

7. Ginther OJ. Reproductive biology of the mare: basic and applied aspects. 2nd edition. Cross Plains (WI): Equiservice; 1992. p. 279–82.

8. Lindholm ARG, Bloemen EHG, Brooks RM, et al. Comparison of deslorelin and buserelin in mares: LH response and induction of ovulation. Anim Reprod Sci 2010;121S:68–70.

9. Macpherson ML, Chaffin MK, Carroll GL, et al. Three methods of oxytocin-induced parturition and their effects of foals. J Am Vet Med Assoc 1997;210: 799–803.

10. Ferris RA, Hatzel JN, Lindholm ARG, et al. Efficacy of Deslorelin acetate (Sucro-Mate) on induction of ovulation in American quarter horse mares. J Equine Vet Sci 2012;32:285–8.

11. Allen WR. Luteal deficiency and embryo mortality in the mare. Reprod Domest Anim 2001;36:121–31.

12. Coffman EA, Pinto CRF, Snyder HK, et al. Antiluteogenic effects of serial prostaglandin F 2α administration in cycling mares. Theriogenology 2014;82:1241–5.

13. Burden CA, McCue PM, Ferris RA. Effect of cloprostenol administration on interval to subsequent ovulation and anovulatory follicle formation in quarter horse mares. J Equine Vet Sci 2015;35:531–5.

14. Vanderwall DK, Rasmussen DM, Woods GL. Effect of repeated administration of oxytocin during diestrus on duration of function of corpora lutea in mares. J Am Vet Med Assoc 2007;231:1864–7.

15. McCue PM, Lemons SS, Squires EL, et al. Efficacy of Synovex-S® implants in suppression of estrus in the mare. J Equine Vet Sci 1997;17:327–9.

16. Stout TAE, Colenbrander B. Suppressing reproductive activity in horses using GnRH vaccines, antagonists or agonists. Anim Reprod Sci 2004;82-83:633–43.

17. Tshewang U, Dowsett KF, Knott LH, et al. Preliminary study of ovarian activity in fillies treated with a GnRH vaccine. Aust Vet J 1997;75:663–7.

18. Tuener RM, Vanderwall DK, Stawicki R. Complications associated with the presence of two intrauterine glass marbles used for oestrus suppression in a mare. Equine Vet Educ 2015;27(7):340–3.

19. Dascanio JJ. Induction of parturition. In: Dascanio J, McCue PM, editors. Equine reproductive procedures manual. Ames (IA): Wiley-Blackwell; 2014. p. 264–6.

20. Duchamp G, Daels PF. Combined effect of sulpiride and light treatment on the onset of cyclicity in anestrous mares. Theriogenology 2002;58:599–602.

21. Meijer M, Macpherson ML, Dijkman R. How to use umbilical vessel water infusion to treat retained fetal membranes in mares. Proceedings Amer Assoc Equine Pract 2015;61:478–84.

22. Allen WR, Wilsher S, Morris L, et al. Laparoscopic application of PGE2 to re-establish oviducal patency and fertility in infertile mares: a preliminary study. Equine Vet J 2006;38:454–9.

Effects of Common Equine Endocrine Diseases on Reproduction

Teresa A. Burns, DVM, PhD

KEYWORDS

- Equine metabolic syndrome (EMS) • Pituitary pars intermedia dysfunction (PPID)
- Fertility • Seasonality • Laminitis • Insulin resistance • Pregnancy • Broodmare

KEY POINTS

- Endocrine diseases, such as equine metabolic syndrome and pituitary pars intermedia dysfunction, are common in domesticated horse populations.
- The frequency with which these diseases are encountered and managed by equine veterinary practitioners is expected to increase as the population ages.
- Equine endocrine diseases have diverse effects on reproductive physiology and fertility, including effects on reproductive seasonality, ovulation efficiency, implantation, early pregnancy loss, duration of pregnancy, and lactation.
- As clinicians learn more about the effects of these diseases on equine reproductive efficiency, strategies and guidelines for how to best improve fertility in affected animals continue to evolve.

INTRODUCTION: EPIDEMIOLOGY AND IMPORTANCE OF EQUINE ENDOCRINE DISEASE
Equine Metabolic Syndrome/Insulin Resistance

The equine metabolic syndrome (EMS), first described in 2002,[1] is perhaps the most common endocrine disorder encountered in equine veterinary practice. The definition of the syndrome is currently held to include obesity (particularly regional adiposity), systemic insulin resistance (IR), and historical or current laminitis.[2] However, this definition is likely ready for refinement based on the research effort that has been directed at characterization of EMS over the past 5 to 10 years; additional characteristics that are likely to be addressed in the case definition in the future include dyslipidemia, hypertension, altered circulating concentrations of biomarkers (including adipokines; eg, leptin and adiponectin), and altered reproductive cyclicity in mares. Subfertility and reproductive failure have been reported to be common in overconditioned equids, but the accompanying pathophysiology linking infertility to obesity in these animals is incompletely characterized to date. Links to human conditions leading to obesity

Equine Internal Medicine, Department of Veterinary Clinical Sciences, The Ohio State University, College of Veterinary Medicine, 601 Vernon L. Tharp St, Columbus, OH 43210, USA
E-mail address: burns.402@osu.edu

Vet Clin Equine 32 (2016) 435–449
http://dx.doi.org/10.1016/j.cveq.2016.07.005
0749-0739/16/© 2016 Elsevier Inc. All rights reserved.

vetequine.theclinics.com

and infertility, such as polycystic ovary syndrome, have been investigated, and although some similarities may exist, substantial species differences exist.

Obesity and its associated metabolic and cardiovascular consequences have emerged over the past 10 to 15 years as critically important conditions in human medicine worldwide, creating a significant economic burden on health care systems of developed nations.[3] In the United States and the United Kingdom, two-thirds of all adults are reported to be either overweight or obese[4–6]; although the magnitude of the obesity epidemic in human populations is well established (and growing), far fewer studies have been performed to describe the epidemiology of obesity and EMS in equids. In addition, most of these studies rely on owner assessments of their horses' body condition and as such may not accurately represent the prevalence of equine obesity. A study of riding horses in Scotland reported that 45% of animals (n = 339) were described by their owners as being fat or very fat,[7] whereas another study from the United Kingdom reported that owners self-reported that their horses were fat or very fat only 17.7% of the time.[8] In the latter study, the owners' assessments were compared with those of an experienced investigator; in this population, owners tended to underscore their horses' body condition score (average by owner = 3.1 out of 5; average by investigator = 3.8 out of 5; k = 0.04). In the United States, the prevalence of equine obesity seems to be similar to that in the United Kingdom (highly prevalent). A study from a general equine veterinary practice population in Virginia reported that, based on the body condition score of 300 horses, 1.7% were underconditioned, 47.3% were of optimal body condition, 32.3% were overweight, and 18.7% were obese.[9] The significance of these high reported prevalence rates for obesity should be underscored, because another cross-sectional study from the United States (central Ohio) investigating risk factors for hyperinsulinemia in light-breed horses reported that obesity was one of only 2 risk factors (along with age) that was significantly associated with hyperinsulinemia in this population.[10] Clearly, obesity is a highly prevalent condition in equids in developed nations (as in humans) and is associated with morbidity in both species.

Pituitary Pars Intermedia Dysfunction

Pituitary pars intermedia dysfunction (PPID; formerly known as equine Cushing's syndrome) is likely the most common endocrinopathy of geriatric equids (>18–20 years of age).[11] The pathophysiology of the condition has been linked to dopaminergic neurodegeneration of hypothalamic neurons within the paraventricular and supraoptic nuclei. Dopaminergic signaling within these neurons results in tonic inhibition of secretory activity of the pars intermedia in health, and loss of this inhibition is thought to result in broadly increased hormone secretion from the pars intermedia in patients with PPID (particularly that of pro-opiomelanocortin-derived peptides), resulting in the pleiotropic and progressive disease phenotype observed in affected individuals.[12] Horses with PPID show a wide variety of clinical signs, but those most frequently reported include hypertrichosis, laminitis, muscle atrophy, hyperhidrosis, weight loss, and polyuria/polydipsia.[13]

To date, no large-scale prospective clinical studies accurately documenting the incidence and prevalence of PPID in domestic equine populations have been performed, and, as such, reported estimates of prevalence of the condition vary widely. However, more limited investigations suggest that conservative estimates make the disease approximately 10 to 15 times more prevalent than Parkinson's disease in humans (another disease that shares common pathophysiology associated with dopaminergic neurodegeneration).[14] A study from the United Kingdom that surveyed owners of horses more than 15 years of age reported that 21.2% of ~340 horses had PPID based on suggestive results of blood tests (endogenous adrenocorticotropic hormone [ACTH], α-melanocyte stimulating hormone concentrations); advanced age and presence of hypertrichosis were associated with increased risk of disease.[15] A practice from the eastern United States reported that ~30% of surveyed horse-owning clients reported hair coat changes in their horses considered highly suggestive of PPID,[16,17] and various postmortem surveys of otherwise normal horses of various ages have documented high prevalence rates of microadenoma or macroadenoma within the pars intermedia at necropsy (30%–40%).[18,19]

DIAGNOSTIC TESTING FOR EQUINE ENDOCRINE DISEASE
Equine Metabolic Syndrome/Insulin Resistance

A diagnosis of EMS can be established based on history (previous bouts of laminitis), clinical signs (body condition score, other measures of adiposity; clinical signs of laminitis; hoof capsule morphology), imaging (pedal radiography), and some laboratory documentation that identifies systemic IR/insulin dysregulation.[20] Many techniques have been described and validated for the assessment of insulin sensitivity in adult horses; however, some tests lend themselves more easily to field use than others. The gold standard tests in equine veterinary medicine for this purpose are the hyperinsulinemic euglycemic clamp method and the frequently sampled insulin-modified intravenous glucose tolerance test (analyzed according to minimal model kinetics); both of these tests give useful information about the degree of insulin dysregulation in horses, but they are highly cumbersome for clinical use.[21] Measurement of basal insulin and glucose concentrations, the oral sugar test (OST), and the combined glucose and insulin test (CGIT) are all more feasible to perform in a hospital or farm setting and can give useful information if performed correctly and interpreted carefully.[20] It is important to keep in mind that these 3 tests (basal insulin, OST, and CGIT) are much more specific than they are sensitive, meaning that normal test results do not rule out IR in any particular patient.[22] Further refinement of these tests (both in test protocol and interpretation parameters) will likely be recommended in the future.

Protocols for assessment of basal insulin concentration, OST, and CGIT are outlined later; the same patient preparation is currently recommended for all tests for IR (access to low non-structural carbohydrate grass hay only for 12 hours pre-test, all feed pulled 2 hours before testing).

Test	Protocol	Interpretation
Basal insulin concentration	Single blood collection in RTT	<20 mIU/L considered normal
OST	Owner administers light corn syrup (15 mL/100 kg PO); blood sample collected in RTT 75 min after dosing for measurement of insulin concentration	Insulin concentration >60 mIU/L suggests IR
CGIT	Measure baseline glucose concentration, then inject 150 mg/kg dextrose IV, followed immediately by 0.1 IU/kg regular insulin; collect blood for glucose concentration at 1, 5, 15, 25, 35, 45, 60, 75, 90, 105, 120, 135, and 150 min after dosing; measure insulin concentration at 45 min after dosing	IR suggested if glucose concentration > baseline value or if insulin concentration >100 mIU/L at 45 min

Abbreviations: IV, intravenous; RTT, red top tube.

Modified from Burns T, Toribio R. Endocrine diseases of the geriatric equid. In: Sprayberry K, Robinson NE, editors. Robinson's current therapy in equine medicine. 7th edition. St. Louis (MO): Elsevier; 2015. p. 582–90.

Pituitary Pars Intermedia Dysfunction

Several diagnostic tests have been evaluated for use in establishing a diagnosis of PPID, with particular interest in the goal of early diagnosis for horses with occult disease. At present, the most commonly recommended diagnostic tests include the endogenous ACTH concentration, the dexamethasone suppression test, and the thyrotropin-releasing hormone (TRH)-stimulation test. Measurement of endogenous adrenocorticotropic hormone (eACTH) concentration in a baseline blood sample is frequently the first-line test of choice, given the simplicity and ease of obtaining the sample (whole blood collected in a plastic purple top tube, chilled immediately, and centrifuged promptly following collection). However, interpretation of the result varies based on the time of year at which the sample is obtained; in the northern hemisphere, values of eACTH concentration greater than 35 pg/mL are consistent with PPID between the months of November and July, whereas from August to October values greater than 100 pg/mL are consistent with the diagnosis. When using seasonally-adjusted reference ranges for eACTH, testing in the autumn months may improve the sensitivity of the test.

Dynamic tests can also be performed and may be more sensitive than baseline eACTH concentration for horses with early disease, particularly when tested during non-autumn months. The TRH-stimulation test is the dynamic test currently recommended by the Equine Endocrinology Group; ideally, this test should be performed between the months of November and July, because reference ranges for interpretation of the result from July to November are currently unavailable.[23] An eACTH concentration greater than 110 pg/mL 10 minutes following the intravenous administration of 1 mg of TRH is consistent with PPID.[23]

EFFECTS OF INSULIN RESISTANCE ON REPRODUCTIVE (OVARIAN) FUNCTION: A HUMAN PERSPECTIVE

Obesity is associated with several common comorbidities in women and men, such as type 2 diabetes mellitus and cardiovascular disease. However, women also frequently develop several reproductive disorders that negatively affect fertility, as well as hormone-responsive neoplasms. IR has been identified as a key risk factor for obesity-related subfertility in women, and there may be several pathophysiologic mechanisms involved. Insulin decreases the production of sex hormone–binding globulin, ultimately resulting in increased (often excessive) ovarian androgen production. This excessive androgen tone represents one of the primary factors leading to abnormal ovarian function and ovulatory disturbances in obese women.[24] Increased leptin concentrations in obese women have also been associated with abnormal ovulation, and this likely occurs not only related to hyperleptinemia's association with IR but also because of direct impairment of normal ovarian function in affected women.[25] Both of these conditions (IR and hyperleptinemia) have been investigated in mares for association with alterations in reproductive efficiency and fertility (described in more detail later).

Polycystic ovary syndrome is one of the most commonly diagnosed endocrine diseases in developed nations and is reported to be the most common cause of infertility/ovarian failure in humans.[24] Similar to the human metabolic syndrome and EMS, the definition of polycystic ovary syndrome has been controversial, because the condition is heterogeneous with sometimes diverse phenotypic presentations. However, most experts agree on the inclusion of the following diagnostic findings in the definition: anovulation with menstrual irregularities, hyperandrogenism, infertility, and metabolic abnormalities (eg, glucose intolerance and dyslipidemia).[24,26] Mares with obesity and

IR have been also been observed to be subfertile, and early analogies were drawn between polycystic ovary syndrome in humans and EMS in obese equidae.[27–31] However, ovarian failure does not seem to play as central a role in the reproductive failure accompanying equine IR as it does in women, because not only do well-conditioned or obese mares show cyclic ovarian activity, many have been reported (anecdotally and in the peer-reviewed literature[29,32]) to cycle year-round and fail to enter seasonal anestrus. Clearly, species differences with respect to the relevant reproductive physiology make direct extrapolation of human information for clinical use in horses and ponies difficult.

EFFECTS OF OBESITY AND INSULIN RESISTANCE ON EQUINE REPRODUCTIVE FUNCTION

The influence of obesity and EMS on concentrations of various hormones of central importance to metabolism and reproductive function in mares has been reported in the veterinary medical literature, although clear practice-changing paradigms have not emerged to date; most conclusions are currently preliminary. Relevant literature pertaining to 2 specific hormones of interest, insulin and leptin, is reviewed here.

Insulin

Horses with EMS are by definition IR and are frequently persistently hyperinsulinemic.[2] Mares with EMS are suspected to have altered reproductive physiology, with some investigators drawing connections between increased serum insulin concentrations and poor fertility. Body condition score and percentage body fat were reported to be inversely correlated with systemic insulin sensitivity and directly (positively) correlated with blood expression levels of interleukin-1 and tumor necrosis factor alpha in mares[31]; these changes were more prominent in older animals, suggesting a relationship between age-related IR and age-related decline in fertility in mares. When mares were rendered transiently IR experimentally through exogenous lipid-heparin infusion, it was associated with increased interovulatory period and higher peak luteal progesterone concentrations.[33] Insulin has also been evaluated as a potential candidate for the signal for equine maternal recognition of pregnancy (MRP); however, after observing that (1) exogenous insulin had no effect on luteal size, diestrus length, interovulatory interval, or circulating luteinizing hormone (LH) concentrations; and (2) insulin was not detected in yolk sac fluid of 32 10-day to 14-day equine conceptuses, the investigators concluded that insulin is unlikely to be the signal of MRP in equids.[34] The role of insulin (and hyperinsulinemia) in the reproductive dysfunction associated with EMS is incompletely characterized, and further work is needed.

Leptin

Leptin is an adipokine produced primarily by white adipose tissue whose blood concentrations have been positively correlated with body condition score and degree of adiposity in many species, including horses. Serum leptin concentration is considered to principally reflect body fat percentage and to be a circulating marker of adiposity (eg, leptin concentration was directly related to body weight in a cohort of Lusitano mares[35]). However, hyperleptinemia is also associated with decreased insulin responsiveness in horses (even when controlling for body condition score[36]), suggesting a direct role for leptin in the pathophysiology of systemic IR.

Overweight or obese mares have been reported to show continuous ovarian cyclicity (ie, fail to enter seasonal anestrus) at a higher rate than lean mares, suggesting a link between nutrition, intermediary metabolism, and reproductive function. Leptin concentrations have been shown to correlate with fat mass, and they also may be altered more acutely by nutrition and medications. Hyperleptinemia was shown to persist across varied management schemes in mares (pasture vs hay in dry lots vs concentrate meal feeding), but the variability in leptin concentrations was minimized when mares were fed hay (which was also associated with minimized variability in insulin and glucose concentrations in the same animals).[37] Feed restriction for as little as 24 hours has been shown to reduce blood leptin concentrations in horses; this change is clearly not associated with a significant reduction in body fat mass.[38] Leptin does not seem to be secreted in a pulsatile fashion in horses, but a circadian rhythm in its concentration has been reported[39]; these investigators also found leptin concentrations to be lower in starved versus fed states, but they additionally reported them to be unaffected by ovariectomy or melatonin implants (obscuring a direct link between leptin and the hypothalamic-pituitary-gonadal axis). This same group later reported that leptin concentrations that have dipped in response to acute feed restriction recover much more slowly than insulin or growth hormone concentrations (which also decrease in response to the same changes in fed state),[40] and although the investigators suggested that diet changes might represent a way to manipulate leptin's effects on reproductive function, subsequent studies suggest that this link is not so direct. Leptin concentrations can also be manipulated pharmacologically, in that exogenous administration of dexamethasone and propylthiouracil were both reported to increase leptin concentrations in mares and geldings after a short period of time.[27,41] Treatment with clenbuterol for 6 months altered body fat and leptin concentrations in light-breed mares in another study, but there was no effect on seasonal anestrus or cyclicity observed in association with these changes.[42]

Because of its connection with nutritional intake and adiposity, leptin has been evaluated as a candidate hormone linking obesity to altered ovarian cyclicity in mares, but the results have been equivocal. One group reported that leptin concentrations were highest in Lipizzan fillies that showed continuous cyclicity and lowest in those that showed seasonal cyclicity, supporting a role for leptin in control of seasonality; concentrations were also highest in the summer months and in older animals in this study.[43] However, in one of the studies referenced earlier,[38] even though acute feed restriction was associated with decreased blood leptin concentrations, it was not associated with concomitant changes in reproductive hormones (prolactin, follicle-stimulating hormone [FSH], LH); this same finding was noted in young and older mares. Although leptin may be responsible for important signaling of metabolic status to the reproductive axis in mares, this signaling likely has to occur over a longer time frame than was evaluated in this study.[38] In another report, leptin and insulin perturbations were not associated with altered ovarian function/cyclicity during winter anestrus and vernal transition.[44] Almost all mares fed to a body condition score of 7.5 to 8.5 in another study showed continuous follicular activity through winter, whereas none of the mares restricted to a body condition score of 3.0 to 3.5 cycled during this time (all went quiescent); leptin concentrations tended to be higher in the overconditioned mares but were highly variable, and no clear relationship with persistent cyclicity could be established in this study.[28,29] Leptin's role in control of reproductive cyclicity in mares remains vague.

Seasonality

The timing of seasonal effects on reproductive cyclicity in horses depends heavily on entrainment by zeitgebers, principally day/photoperiod length, and this timing of annual reproductive rhythms is driven by melatonin secretion by the pineal gland. Seasonality (especially the occurrence and length of seasonal anestrus) has been shown to be controlled to some extent by metabolic hormones and correlated with body condition. Older mares were more likely to not undergo seasonal anestrus and to enter it later than younger mares in one study; the investigators reported that propensity for continuous cycling was associated with body condition, body fat percentage, and serum leptin concentration (all of which were highest in summer months).[45] Welsh pony mares (a breed likely to be more relevant to a discussion of IR and EMS than many light breeds[46]) fed to low body condition scores always showed seasonal anestrus, which persisted longer than in mares that were well fed (only 40% of these mares showed seasonal anestrus, which was shorter than in other groups).[32] Large differences in growth hormone, insulin-like growth factor-1, and leptin concentrations were observed between the well-fed and restricted groups, and glucose, insulin, growth hormone, and leptin levels were highly correlated with duration of ovulatory activity.[32] However, in a population of mares not predisposed to IR/EMS, flushing (ie, acute increase in plane of nutrition, body condition score, and body fat percentage ~3 weeks before the breeding season) stimulated ovarian activity in stressed maiden Standardbred mares (and presumably improved their reproductive efficiency)[47]; hormonal activities were not evaluated in this study, simply time to first seasonal ovulation (which was minimized in mares in better body condition).

Little information exists regarding the role of plane of nutrition and endocrine disease status on reproductive performance during pregnancy and lactation in horses. Kubiak and colleagues[48] showed that feeding mares to obesity during gestation had no detectable effect on postpartum reproductive performance (times to first and second postfoaling ovulation, conception rates, and early pregnancy loss rates were similar to those of mares maintained at a moderate body condition score). Even a high degree of body fat produced by overfeeding during gestation did not seem to adversely affect postpartum reproductive performance in multiparous mares.[48] Anecdotally, foals may have difficulty nursing (at least initially) from overconditioned mares that accumulate excessive adipose tissue within or near their mammary glands, which can efface the teats and make them less prominent. In addition, mares with historical or current endocrinopathic laminitis may experience increased orthopedic pain that is difficult to control as they gain weight during the third trimester of pregnancy. Even if reproductive efficiency does not decrease directly because of increased adiposity, these would represent good reasons to maintain ideal body condition in broodmares (during and after/before pregnancy).

In addition, in other species, robust evidence supports a role for maternal nutrition and metabolism in the programming of future metabolic pathways of the offspring while still in utero. Although fetal macrosomia is a common complication in children born to women with IR and diabetes mellitus (gestational or otherwise), children born prematurely to affected mothers (although initially often reported to have intrauterine growth restriction and low birth weight), later have significantly increased risk of obesity, IR, and type II diabetes mellitus in adulthood. Evidence for gestational programming in horses is lacking, but a few studies have investigated links between maternal and fetal/neonatal metabolism in this species. Leptin concentrations in nursing mares were shown not to affect leptin, triglyceride, or free fatty acid concentrations in their foals,[49] but maternal nutritional restriction during midgestation was associated with altered pancreatic responsiveness following birth in their (otherwise normal) foals.[50] Mid-gestational maternal nutritional restriction was associated with an increased acute insulin response to glucose (enhanced pancreatic β-cell responsiveness) in the neonates, although no differences in response to ACTH stimulation or exogenous insulin administration was observed in foals from high-condition mares compared with those in moderate condition.[50] The long-term significance of these findings remains to be determined, but this preliminary evidence for gestational metabolic programming in horses may represent the best reason for maintaining the endocrine health of broodmares; the strength of this recommendation awaits support from additional studies.

Medical management of broodmares with equine metabolic syndrome/insulin resistance

Optimization of diet and exercise, as well as management of endocrinopathic laminitis if present, are the mainstays of treatment of horses and ponies with EMS; the same strategies that are recommended for the general equine population can also be used for managing affected broodmares, particularly in the first and second trimesters of gestation (when metabolic demands and weight gain are not yet significantly different from the nongravid state). These strategies may be appropriate for most broodmares, because IR is physiologic and progressive during normal pregnancy (this would be expected to be enhanced, and more likely pathologic, in animals with pre-pregnancy EMS). Provision of a diet primarily composed of grass hay, ideally shown to contain less than 10% non-structural carbohydrate on a dry matter basis through forage analysis, and some sort of ration balancer to ensure adequate trace mineral and vitamin intake are central to dietary management of EMS cases; nutritional goals include minimizing dietary non-structural carbohydrate (sugars, starches, and fructans) and encouraging safe, gradual weight loss if needed (the timing and rate of weight loss that is appropriate and safe for broodmares is currently unclear, but prevention of excessive weight gain during gestation seems to be a reasonable goal in this population). Continuous consumption of forage is considered ideal for horses and ponies in general, but the timing of feeding was recently shown to affect fertility in mares.[51] Mares with continuous access to forage showed higher rates of fertility and fewer estrus abnormalities than mares offered forage only at night. Continuous forage access may be important for maximizing fertility in broodmares in general, but particularly those who may have dietary restriction as a part of a treatment plan for EMS/IR. During the third trimester of gestation and onset of lactation, most broodmares require supplemental calories in the form of concentrate to maintain body weight and support these increased metabolic demands; the composition of that concentrate can affect insulin sensitivity of the mare, even in the absence of a significant change in body weight or composition. A study comparing the effects of dietary composition on insulin sensitivity in broodmares showed that provision of a diet rich in sugar and starch enhanced IR compared with forage only or a fat-and-fiber-rich diet; this effect was enhanced in mares with higher body condition scores.[52] The investigators recommended using fat-and-fiber-rich diets to provide supplemental calories in broodmares, in addition to avoiding overweight or obesity in this population; this recommendation seems particularly salient, considering what is now known in horses and other species about gestational metabolic programming.[53–57]

The effects of exercise and pharmaceuticals on management of EMS and IR in broodmares have not been investigated, but these strategies may be useful as well. Exercise in particular may prove highly valuable, because it is likely to be safe (at least in the first and second trimesters, and as long as the animal is sound and comfortable), inexpensive, and highly effective in improving insulin sensitivity both acutely following an exercise bout and chronically in conjunction with weight loss and improvement in body composition. As little as 30 minutes of trot exercise daily is useful, because this amount of exercise has been shown to elicit improvement in insulin sensitivity in the absence of any change in body condition or body weight in both lean and obese (albeit nonpregnant) mares[58]; this benefit was observed almost immediately following institution of the exercise program, but it did not persist long past discontinuation of the protocol. Consistency, therefore seems to be important to maximize the benefits achieved from an exercise plan.

Regarding pharmaceutical use in the management of broodmares with EMS, there are no studies of safety or efficacy of medications such as levothyroxine or metformin in pregnant equids. Based on the known risks to the fetus associated with maternal hyperthyroidism in humans,[59–61] the empiric safety of levothyroxine use during equine pregnancy should not be assumed. The efficacy of metformin in improving IR in horses remains to be characterized more fully, but the drug seems to be reasonably safe in horses.[62] Metformin has not been evaluated for safety in pregnant mares, but this drug is frequently used in diabetic pregnant women with an excellent safety profile.[63] If diet and exercise fail to achieve therapeutic goals in an at-risk pregnant mare, metformin treatment may be warranted.

EFFECTS OF PITUITARY PARS INTERMEDIA DYSFUNCTION ON EQUINE REPRODUCTIVE FUNCTION

As equine populations age, and as horse owners maintain the health of their animals well into their third (and fourth) decades, the number of middle-aged and geriatric horses presented for reproductive management will undoubtedly increase. Mares can conceive and carry foals well into their third decade, and this will occur more commonly as management and medical progress increase the number of geriatric animals attended by many equine veterinary practices. Aged mares are more likely to require veterinary management for fertility issues; in one study, increasing age of mares was the greatest limiting factor for reproductive performance in flat race and National Hunt thoroughbreds in the United Kingdom.[64] In another study that evaluated the reproductive performance of 1482 thoroughbred broodmares mated to 2 stallions on a well-managed farm across 3 consecutive breeding seasons, investigators identified 2 primary factors associated with reproductive performance: mare age and foaling status. Increasing age was associated with significantly reduced reproductive performance regardless of foaling status, and foaling mares had a significantly poorer reproductive performance compared with dry mares controlled for age. More than 90% of the variation in reproductive performance in this study was at the mare level (compared with stallion influence [4%–6%] and farm influence [0%–1%]).[65] Another group evaluated 430 mares mated to 2 thoroughbred stallions on a well-managed farm, and they reported that the age of the mares had a significant adverse effect on live foal rates, with mares greater than 13 years of age having a lower rate than younger mares. Resorption and abortion occurred in higher percentages among mares greater than 8 years of age, and the investigators concluded that age of mares was associated with decreased reproductive efficiency.[66] Even in the absence of a direct adverse effect of PPID on mare reproductive performance, affected broodmares are likely to require veterinary management for an expected age-related decline in fertility; veterinarians are likely to encounter these mares with increasing frequency in the future, making knowledge of PPID testing and treatment that much more relevant and important.

Although the effects of PPID on equine reproductive performance have not been evaluated in great depth to date, it seems reasonable to assume that there should be influence, given the pathophysiology of the disease as it is currently understood. The pars intermedia is involved in regulation of certain seasonal functions in equids (eg, growing and shedding of the hair coat), and the seasonality of equine reproduction has also long been recognized; initial evidence was presented in 1979 that the pineal-hypothalamopituitary axis influences annual seasonal patterns of reproductive activity in horses.[67] The effects of cortisol and related metabolites on reproductive hormone secretion have long been held to negatively affect fertility; however, horses with PPID are inconsistently hypercortisolemic,[68] and work by Berghold and colleagues[69] suggests that, even when cortisol secretion is high, effects on subsequent fertility are minimal (mares diagnosed with PPID were not specifically evaluated in this study).

Dopaminergic neurodegeneration in certain subsets of hypothalamic neurons has been implicated as directly involved in the pathogenesis of PPID,[12] and pergolide, a dopaminergic agonist, is currently the recommended treatment of the disease. The role of dopamine in control of reproductive cyclicity in mares has been evaluated (albeit in otherwise normal mares, not those with PPID).[70] Suppression of dopaminergic activity via treatment of normal mares with sulpiride (a D2 antagonist) during seasonal anestrus resulted in advancement of the mean day of first seasonal ovulation in mares managed under conditions of natural photoperiod. Plasma prolactin concentrations were also increased 2 and 9 hours after sulpiride administration, returning to baseline levels by 24 hours. Concentrations of LH and FSH were also higher in mares treated with sulpiride at the time of first ovulation than in untreated mares. The investigators concluded that dopamine plays a role in the control of reproductive seasonality in mares and exerts a tonic inhibition on reproductive activity during the anovulatory season.[70] This finding suggests that although mares with PPID may cycle regularly (and they may be more likely to cycle for a greater part of the year than normal mares; pharmacologic inhibition of dopaminergic neurotransmission resulted in increased follicular development and plasma estrogen and prolactin concentrations in mares in one study[71]), effective treatment of PPID in the form of dopaminergic agonists may then adversely affect cyclicity. Moreover, this treatment is likely to suppress prolactin secretion (protocols for induction of lactation in mares have been described using dopaminergic antagonists[72,73]), suggesting that hypogalactia and agalactia are more likely to be problematic in lactating mares with PPID.[71]

Medical Management of Broodmares with Pituitary Pars Intermedia Dysfunction

Treatment of horses with PPID involves administration of medication to suppress secretory activity of the pars intermedia (the current US Food and Drug Administration–approved drug of choice is pergolide, a dopaminergic agonist) and management changes.[12] In pregnant and lactating animals, pergolide administration may increase the risk of prolonged gestation, premature placental separation, and hypogalactia/agalactia. It may be appropriate in this case to manage PPID-affected mares according to established recommendations for mares at risk for ergot alkaloid exposure from grazing endophyte-infested fescue pasture during gestation (also a condition linked to dopamine agonism[74–76]); strategies such as temporary discontinuation of pergolide therapy 30 days before the expected foaling date and judicious use of dopaminergic antagonists such as domperidone or sulpiride may be useful for prevention of prolonged gestation and for encouraging normal lactation.[77,78] Mares should be monitored after foaling to ensure that they have adequate milk production; poor foal growth and incessant/continuous nursing on the part of the foal suggest that milk production may be inadequate, and supplementation with milk replacer, goat's milk, and/or a milk-based creep feed may be warranted. Pergolide therapy is often reinstituted at approximately 30 days after foaling; if the mare's PPID is poorly controlled without medication, she should likely receive treatment sooner than this, and alternative sources of nutrition for the foal may be required (including the option of a nurse mare). Alternatively, affected mares that do not tolerate withdrawal of medication at all may be used most effectively as embryo donors if their genetics are sufficiently valuable; however, pergolide treatment would be expected to decrease the efficiency of oocyte and/or embryo collection from these mares. Further work to optimize assisted reproduction protocols for mares with PPID is needed to guide best practice.

Although not all horses with PPID have systemic IR,[79] this is a common finding in this population.[80] Provision of sufficient calories to support lactation in insulin-resistant horses (particularly those that have recently had a bout of laminitis) requires careful attention to the composition of the diet to avoid inciting complications associated with hyperinsulinemia.[81,82] Feedstuffs with calories primarily coming from fat and fermentable fiber should be offered, and sugars, starches, and fructans in the diet should be minimized as much as possible. Body condition of affected mares should be carefully maintained within a normal range (4.5–6.5 on the Henneke scale[83]) to ensure sufficient reserves to support lactation and avoid overconditioning (excessive body weight is expected to complicate clinical laminitis, particularly in late gestation when the mare's weight is already substantially increased). With careful implementation and monitoring of diet, medication, and management modifications, broodmares with PPID can continue to be healthy and productive well into their third decade of life.

SUMMARY

Endocrine diseases, such as EMS and PPID, are common in domesticated horse populations, and the frequency with which these diseases are encountered and managed by equine veterinary practitioners is expected to increase as the population ages. As clinicians learn more about the effects of these diseases on equine reproductive physiology and efficiency (including effects on reproductive seasonality, ovulation efficiency, implantation, early pregnancy loss, duration of pregnancy, and lactation), strategies and guidelines for how to best improve fertility in affected animals continue to evolve. It is hoped that further research will establish more firmly the evidence base on which these recommendations are based.

REFERENCES

1. Johnson PJ. The equine metabolic syndrome peripheral Cushing's syndrome. Vet Clin North Am Equine Pract 2002;18(2):271–93.
2. Frank N, Geor RJ, Bailey SR, et al, American College of Veterinary Internal Medicine. Equine metabolic syndrome. J Vet Intern Med 2010;24(3):467–75.
3. Polonsky KS. The past 200 years in diabetes. N Engl J Med 2012;367(14):1332–40.
4. Ljungvall A, Zimmerman FJ. Bigger bodies: long-term trends and disparities in obesity and body-mass index among U.S. adults, 1960-2008. Soc Sci Med 2012;75(1):109–19.
5. Martinson ML. Income inequality in health at all ages: a comparison of the United States and England. Am J Public Health 2012;102(11):2049–56.
6. Stevens VL, Jacobs EJ, Sun J, et al. Weight cycling and mortality in a large prospective US study. Am J Epidemiol 2012;175(8):785–92.
7. Wyse CA, McNie KA, Tannahill VJ, et al. Prevalence of obesity in riding horses in Scotland. Vet Rec 2008;162(18):590–1.
8. Stephenson HM, Green MJ, Freeman SL. Prevalence of obesity in a population of horses in the UK. Vet Rec 2011;168(5):131.
9. Thatcher CD, Pleasant RS, Geor RJ, et al. Prevalence of overconditioning in mature horses in southwest Virginia during the summer. J Vet Intern Med 2012;26(6):1413–8.

10. Muno J, Gallatin L, Geor RJ, et al. Research Abstract Program of the 2009 ACVIM Forum and Canadian Veterinary Medical Association Convention. Abstract #124. Journal of Veterinary Internal Medicine 2009;23(3):721.

11. Burns T, Toribio R. Endocrine diseases of the geriatric equid. In: Sprayberry K, Robinson NE, editors. Robinson's current therapy in equine medicine. 7th edition. St. Louis (MO): Elsevier; 2015. p. 582–90.

12. McFarlane D. Equine pituitary pars intermedia dysfunction. Vet Clin North Am Equine Pract 2011;27(1):93–113.

13. Rohrbach BW, Stafford JR, Clermont RS, et al. Diagnostic frequency, response to therapy, and long-term prognosis among horses and ponies with pituitary par intermedia dysfunction, 1993-2004. J Vet Intern Med 2012;26(4):1027–34.

14. McFarlane D. Advantages and limitations of the equine disease, pituitary pars intermedia dysfunction as a model of spontaneous dopaminergic neurodegenerative disease. Ageing Res Rev 2007;6(1):54–63.

15. McGowan TW, Pinchbeck GP, McGowan CM. Prevalence, risk factors and clinical signs predictive for equine pituitary pars intermedia dysfunction in aged horses. Equine Vet J 2013;45(1):74–9.

16. Brosnahan MM, Paradis MR. Assessment of clinical characteristics, management practices, and activities of geriatric horses. J Am Vet Med Assoc 2003;223(1):99–103.

17. Brosnahan MM, Paradis MR. Demographic and clinical characteristics of geriatric horses: 467 cases (1989-1999). J Am Vet Med Assoc 2003;223(1):93–8.

18. van der Kolk JH, Heinrichs M, van Amerongen JD, et al. Evaluation of pituitary gland anatomy and histopathologic findings in clinically normal horses and horses and ponies with pituitary pars intermedia adenoma. Am J Vet Res 2004;65(12):1701–7.

19. Frank N, Andrews FM, Sommardahl CS, et al. Evaluation of the combined dexamethasone suppression/thyrotropin-releasing hormone stimulation test for detection of pars intermedia pituitary adenomas in horses. J Vet Intern Med 2006;20(4):987–93.

20. Frank N. Equine metabolic syndrome. Vet Clin North Am Equine Pract 2011;27(1):73–92.

21. Firshman AM, Valberg SJ. Factors affecting clinical assessment of insulin sensitivity in horses. Equine Vet J 2007;39(6):567–75.

22. Dunbar LK, Mielnicki KA, Dembek KA, et al. Evaluation of four diagnostic tests for insulin dysregulation in adult light-breed horses. J Vet Intern Med 2016;30(3):885–91.

23. Frank N, Andrews F, Durham A, et al. Recommendations for the diagnosis and treatment of pituitary pars intermedia dysfunction (PPID). Equine Endocrinology Group; 2015.

24. Ehrmann DA. Polycystic ovary syndrome. N Engl J Med 2005;352(12):1223–36.

25. Pasquali R, Gambineri A. Metabolic effects of obesity on reproduction. Reprod Biomed Online 2006;12(5):542–51.

26. Trikudanathan S. Polycystic ovarian syndrome. Med Clin North Am 2015;99(1):221–35.

27. Cartmill JA, Thompson DL Jr, Storer WA, et al. Endocrine responses in mares and geldings with high body condition scores grouped by high vs. low resting leptin concentrations. J Anim Sci 2003;81(9):2311–21.

28. Gentry LR, Thompson DL Jr, Gentry GT Jr, et al. High versus low body condition in mares: interactions with responses to somatotropin, GnRH analog, and dexamethasone. J Anim Sci 2002;80(12):3277–85.

29. Gentry LR, Thompson DL Jr, Gentry GT Jr, et al. The relationship between body condition, leptin, and reproductive and hormonal characteristics of mares during the seasonal anovulatory period. J Anim Sci 2002;80(10):2695–703.

30. Vick MM, Sessions DR, Murphy BA, et al. Obesity is associated with altered metabolic and reproductive activity in the mare: effects of metformin on insulin sensitivity and reproductive cyclicity. Reprod Fertil Dev 2006;18(6):609–17.

31. Vick MM, Adams AA, Murphy BA, et al. Relationships among inflammatory cytokines, obesity, and insulin sensitivity in the horse. J Anim Sci 2007;85(5):1144–55.

32. Salazar-Ortiz J, Camous S, Briant C, et al. Effects of nutritional cues on the duration of the winter anovulatory phase and on associated hormone levels in adult female Welsh pony horses (*Equus caballus*). Reprod Biol Endocrinol 2011;9:130.

33. Sessions DR, Reedy SE, Vick MM, et al. Development of a model for inducing transient insulin resistance in the mare: preliminary implications regarding the estrous cycle. J Anim Sci 2004;82(8):2321–8.

34. Rambags BP, van Rossem AW, Blok EE, et al. Effects of exogenous insulin on luteolysis and reproductive cyclicity in the mare. Reprod Domest Anim 2008;43(4): 422–8.

35. Ferreira-Dias G, Claudino F, Carvalho H, et al. Seasonal reproduction in the mare: possible role of plasma leptin, body weight and immune status. Domest Anim Endocrinol 2005;29(1):203–13.

36. Caltabilota TJ, Earl LR, Thompson DL Jr, et al. Hyperleptinemia in mares and geldings: assessment of insulin sensitivity from glucose responses to insulin injection. J Anim Sci 2010;88(9):2940–9.

37. Storer WA, Thompson DL Jr, Waller CA, et al. Hormonal patterns in normal and hyperleptinemic mares in response to three common feeding-housing regimens. J Anim Sci 2007;85(11):2873–81.

38. McManus CJ, Fitzgerald BP. Effects of a single day of feed restriction on changes in serum leptin, gonadotropins, prolactin, and metabolites in aged and young mares. Domest Anim Endocrinol 2000;19(1):1–13.

39. Buff PR, Morrison CD, Ganjam VK, et al. Effects of short-term feed deprivation and melatonin implants on circadian patterns of leptin in the horse. J Anim Sci 2005;83(5):1023–32.

40. Buff PR, Spader BR, Morrison CD, et al. Endocrine responses in mares undergoing abrupt changes in nutritional management. J Anim Sci 2006;84(10):2700–7.

41. Cartmill JA, Thompson DL Jr, Gentry LR, et al. Effects of dexamethasone, glucose infusion, adrenocorticotropin, and propylthiouracil on plasma leptin concentrations in horses. Domest Anim Endocrinol 2003;24(1):1–14.

42. Fitzgerald BP, Reedy SE, Sessions DR, et al. Potential signals mediating the maintenance of reproductive activity during the non-breeding season of the mare. Reprod Suppl 2002;59:115–29.

43. Cebulj-Kadunc N, Kosec M, Cestnik V. Serum leptin concentrations in Lipizzan fillies. Reprod Domest Anim 2009;44(1):1–5.

44. Waller CA, Thompson DL Jr, Cartmill JA, et al. Reproduction in high body condition mares with high versus low leptin concentrations. Theriogenology 2006; 66(4):923–8.

45. Fitzgerald BP, McManus CJ. Photoperiodic versus metabolic signals as determinants of seasonal anestrus in the mare. Biol Reprod 2000;63(1):335–40.

46. Treiber KH, Kronfeld DS, Hess TM, et al. Evaluation of genetic and metabolic predispositions and nutritional risk factors for pasture-associated laminitis in ponies. J Am Vet Med Assoc 2006;228(10):1538–45.

47. Vecchi I, Sabbioni A, Bigliardi E, et al. Relationship between body fat and body condition score and their effects on estrous cycles of the standardbred maiden mare. Vet Res Commun 2010;34(Suppl 1):S41–5.

48. Kubiak JR, Evans JW, Potter GD, et al. Postpartum reproductive performance in the multiparous mare fed to obesity. Theriogenology 1989;32(1):27–36.

49. Kedzierski W, Kusy R, Kowalik S. Plasma leptin level in hyperlipidemic mares and their newborn foals. Reprod Domest Anim 2011;46(2):275–80.

50. Ousey JC, Fowden AL, Wilsher S, et al. The effects of maternal health and body condition on the endocrine responses of neonatal foals. Equine Vet J 2008;40(7): 673–9.

51. Benhajali H, Ezzaouia M, Lunel C, et al. Temporal feeding pattern may influence reproduction efficiency, the example of breeding mares. PLoS One 2013;8(9): e73858.

52. Hoffman RM, Kronfeld DS, Cooper WL, et al. Glucose clearance in grazing mares is affected by diet, pregnancy, and lactation. J Anim Sci 2003;81(7):1764–71.

53. Desai M, Jellyman JK, Ross MG. Epigenomics, gestational programming and risk of metabolic syndrome. Int J Obes (Lond) 2015;39(4):633–41.

54. Ojha S, Fainberg HP, Sebert S, et al. Maternal health and eating habits: metabolic consequences and impact on child health. Trends Mol Med 2015;21(2):126–33.

55. Rodriguez L, Panadero MI, Roglans N, et al. Fructose only in pregnancy provokes hyperinsulinemia, hypoadiponectinemia, and impaired insulin signaling in adult male, but not female, progeny. Eur J Nutr 2016;55(2):665–74.

56. Sipola-Leppanen M, Vaarasmaki M, Tikanmaki M, et al. Cardiometabolic risk factors in young adults who were born preterm. Am J Epidemiol 2015;181(11): 861–73.

57. Smith CJ, Ryckman KK. Epigenetic and developmental influences on the risk of obesity, diabetes, and metabolic syndrome. Diabetes Metab Syndr Obes 2015;8: 295–302.

58. Powell DM, Reedy SE, Sessions DR, et al. Effect of short-term exercise training on insulin sensitivity in obese and lean mares. Equine Vet J Suppl 2002;(34):81–4.

59. Sheehan PM, Nankervis A, Araujo Junior E, et al. Maternal thyroid disease and preterm birth: systematic review and meta-analysis. J Clin Endocrinol Metab 2015;100(11):4325–31.

60. Spencer L, Bubner T, Bain E, et al. Screening and subsequent management for thyroid dysfunction pre-pregnancy and during pregnancy for improving maternal and infant health. Cochrane Database Syst Rev 2015;(9):CD011263.

61. van der Kaay DC, Wasserman JD, Palmert MR. Management of neonates born to mothers with Graves' disease. Pediatrics 2016;137(4) [pii peds.2015-1878].

62. Durham AE, Rendle DI, Newton JE. The effect of metformin on measurements of insulin sensitivity and beta cell response in 18 horses and ponies with insulin resistance. Equine Vet J 2008;40(5):493–500.

63. Rowan JA, Hague WM, Gao W, et al. MiG Trial Investigators. Metformin versus insulin for the treatment of gestational diabetes. N Engl J Med 2008;358(19): 2003–15.

64. Allen WR, Brown L, Wright M, et al. Reproductive efficiency of flatrace and National Hunt thoroughbred mares and stallions in England. Equine Vet J 2007; 39(5):438–45.

65. Hanlon DW, Stevenson M, Evans MJ, et al. Reproductive performance of thoroughbred mares in the Waikato region of New Zealand: 2. Multivariable analyses and sources of variation at the mare, stallion and stud farm level. N Z Vet J 2012; 60(6):335–43.

66. Hemberg E, Lundeheim N, Einarsson S. Reproductive performance of thoroughbred mares in Sweden. Reprod Domest Anim 2004;39(2):81–5.
67. Sharp DC, Vernon MW, Zavy MT. Alteration of seasonal reproductive patterns in mares following superior cervical ganglionectomy. J Reprod Fertil Suppl 1979;(27):87–93.
68. Haritou SJ, Zylstra R, Ralli C, et al. Seasonal changes in circadian peripheral plasma concentrations of melatonin, serotonin, dopamine and cortisol in aged horses with Cushing's disease under natural photoperiod. J Neuroendocrinol 2008;20(8):988–96.
69. Berghold P, Mostl E, Aurich C. Effects of reproductive status and management on cortisol secretion and fertility of oestrous horse mares. Anim Reprod Sci 2007; 102(3–4):276–85.
70. Besognet B, Hansen BS, Daels PF. Induction of reproductive function in anestrous mares using a dopamine antagonist. Theriogenology 1997;47(2):467–80.
71. Brendemuehl JP, Cross DL. Influence of the dopamine antagonist domperidone on the vernal transition in seasonally anoestrous mares. J Reprod Fertil Suppl 2000;(56):185–93.
72. Guillaume D, Chavatte-Palmer P, Combarnous Y, et al. Induced lactation with a dopamine antagonist in mares: different responses between ovariectomized and intact mares. Reprod Domest Anim 2003;38(5):394–400.
73. Chavatte-Palmer P, Arnaud G, Duvaux-Ponter C, et al. Quantitative and qualitative assessment of milk production after pharmaceutical induction of lactation in the mare. J Vet Intern Med 2002;16(4):472–7.
74. Blodgett DJ. Fescue toxicosis. Vet Clin North Am Equine Pract 2001;17(3): 567–77.
75. Evans TJ. Endocrine alterations associated with ergopeptine alkaloid exposure during equine pregnancy. Vet Clin North Am Equine Pract 2002;18(2):371–8, viii.
76. McCann JS, Caudle AB, Thompson FN, et al. Influence of endophyte-infected tall fescue on serum prolactin and progesterone in gravid mares. J Anim Sci 1992; 70(1):217–23.
77. Cross DL, Reinemeyer CR, Prado JC, et al. Efficacy of domperidone gel in an induced model of fescue toxicosis in periparturient mares. Theriogenology 2012;78(6):1361–70.
78. Redmond LM, Cross DL, Strickland JR, et al. Efficacy of domperidone and sulpiride as treatments for fescue toxicosis in horses. Am J Vet Res 1994;55(5):722–9.
79. Mastro LM, Adams AA, Urschel KL. Pituitary pars intermedia dysfunction does not necessarily impair insulin sensitivity in old horses. Domest Anim Endocrinol 2015;50:14–25.
80. Klinkhamer K, Menheere PP, van der Kolk JH. Basal glucose metabolism and peripheral insulin sensitivity in equine pituitary pars intermedia dysfunction. Vet Q 2011;31(1):19–28.
81. Asplin KE, Sillence MN, Pollitt CC, et al. Induction of laminitis by prolonged hyperinsulinaemia in clinically normal ponies. Vet J 2007;174(3):530–5.
82. de Laat MA, McGowan CM, Sillence MN, et al. Equine laminitis: induced by 48 h hyperinsulinaemia in standardbred horses. Equine Vet J 2010;42(2):129–35.
83. Henneke DR, Potter GD, Kreider JL, et al. Relationship between condition score, physical measurements and body fat percentage in mares. Equine Vet J 1983; 15(4):371–2.

Biological Functions and Clinical Applications of Anti-Müllerian Hormone in Stallions and Mares

Anthony N.J. Claes, DVM, PhD[a],*, Barry A. Ball, DVM, PhD[b]

KEYWORDS

- Anti-Müllerian hormone • Equine • Mare • Stallion • Cryptorchidism
- Sertoli cell tumor • Ovarian reserve • Equine granulosa cell tumor

KEY POINTS

- Anti-Müllerian hormone (AMH) can serve as an endocrine marker for equine cryptorchidism and as an immunohistochemical marker for Sertoli cell tumors.
- AMH can be useful in the assessment of ovarian reserve and reproductive life-span of aged mares.
- AMH can serve as a diagnostic marker for equine granulosa cell tumors.

BASIC ASPECTS OF ANTI-MÜLLERIAN HORMONE
The Discovery of Anti-Müllerian Hormone

The discovery of anti-Müllerian hormone (AMH) dates back to the middle of last century when Alfred Jost, a French physiologist, was interested in the process of sexual differentiation. Initially, he showed that when fetal gonads were removed in utero (**Fig. 1**, top right), the Müllerian or paramesonephric ducts developed and the Wolffian of mesonephric ducts regressed.[1] Consequently, it was assumed that testosterone plays a key role in sexual differentiation; this was rejected because administration of androgens to female fetuses (see **Fig. 1**, bottom right) resulted in differentiation of the Wolffian ducts while the Müllerian ducts failed to regress. However, when small pieces of testicular tissue were grafted in close proximity to the ovary (see **Fig. 1**, bottom left), regression of Müllerian ducts was observed, indicating that the fetal testis must have an important role in sexual differentiation. Therefore, Alfred Jost concluded that the fetal testis does not only produce androgens, but also secretes another

[a] Department of Equine Science, Faculty of Veterinary Medicine, Utrecht University, Yalelaan 114, Utrecht 3584 CM, The Netherlands; [b] Department of Veterinary Science, Gluck Equine Research Center, University of Kentucky, 1400 Nicholasville Road, Lexington, KY, 40546-0099 USA
* Corresponding author.
E-mail address: a.claes@uu.nl

Vet Clin Equine 32 (2016) 451–464
http://dx.doi.org/10.1016/j.cveq.2016.07.004
0749-0739/16/© 2016 Elsevier Inc. All rights reserved.

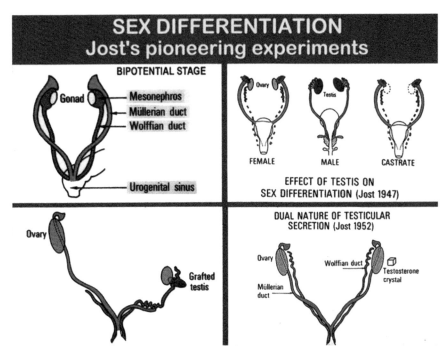

Fig. 1. Pioneering experiments conducted by Alfred Jost who investigated the underlying mechanism of sexual differentiation. (*Top left*) Internal reproductive organs prior to sexual differentiation (bipotential stage). (*Top right*) Removal of the fetal gonads in utero resulted in regression of the Wolffian of mesonephric ducts while the Müllerian or paramesonephric ducts developed. (*Bottom right*) Administration of androgens to female fetuses resulted in differentiation of the Wolffian ducts while the Müllerian ducts failed to regress. (*Bottom left*) Grafting small pieces of testicular tissue in close proximity to the ovary resulted in regression of Müllerian ducts indicating that the fetal testis must have an important role in sexual differentiation. (*From* Rey R, Josso N. Sexual differentiation. In: de Groot LJ, Beck-Peccoz P, Chrousos G, et al, editors. Endotext. South Dartmouth (MA): MDText.com, Inc; 2000; with permission from MDText.com, Inc.)

substance that induces the regression of the Müllerian ducts.[2] Although the nature of this substance remained unidentified, he defined it as 'hormone inhibitrice,' which later became better known as the Müllerian-inhibiting substance, Müllerian-inhibiting factor, or AMH.[3]

Anti-Müllerian Hormone: The Protein

Although the existence of a substance 'hormone inhibitrice' was already implied by Alfred Jost in 1953,[2] specific information about this substance remained unknown for some time. One of the first studies examining AMH indicated that it was a large molecule, such as a polypeptide, because it was not able pass through a membrane that allowed the passage of androgens.[4] Subsequent experiments demonstrated that AMH was a glycoprotein,[5,6] which contained disulfide bridges as smaller fragments were obtained when preparations of fetal testes were examined using sodium dodecyl sulfate polyacrylamide gel electrophoresis under reducing conditions.[6] As the methods of AMH purification improved, more detailed information was obtained about the physical properties of this glycoprotein[7] as well as its biochemical composition with respect to amino acids and carbohydrates.[8,9] The protein AMH is derived from a precursor that varies slightly in length among different species, ranging from 553 (rat) to 575 (bovine) amino acids.[3] The equine precursor is similar to the length of the bovine precursor with 573 amino acids (unpublished data, Drs Ball and Conley; National Center for Biotechnology Information: GenBank AEA11205.1, 2012). The amino acid sequence of the carboxyl terminal portion of the precursor is highly conserved across different species and among other members of the transforming growth factor-β family. In contrast, the amino acid sequence in the amino-terminal region is less conserved between different species.[3] Furthermore, the bovine AMH precursor starts with a signal sequence (16–17 amino acids) followed by a prosequence (7–8 amino acids). However, both sequences are cleaved from the precursor before secretion.[9] Finally, dimerization of the remaining monomer (70 kDa) results in the formation of the glycoprotein AMH, which is approximately 140 kDa.[10] Another interesting feature of this 140 kDa AMH glycoprotein is that cleavage is not required for it to be biologically active. Nonetheless, in vitro cleavage of AMH using plasmin also results in a biologically active product, which contains a 25-kDa and 110-kDa fragment representing the carboxyl and amino terminal dimer, respectively. Furthermore, sequencing of those fragments revealed that cleavage occurs at the monobasic cleavage site between the amino acid arginine and serine; 109 amino acids upstream of the carboxyl terminus.[11] Interestingly, the biological activity of AMH is localized in carboxyl terminal fragment while the amino terminal fragment is biologically inactive.[12] However, even though this amino terminal fragment is biologically inactive by itself, it supports the activity of the carboxyl terminal fragment because more complete regression of Müllerian ducts is observed when both fragments are included in organ culture media compared with only the carboxyl terminal fragment.[13]

Anti-Müllerian Hormone: The Gene

In 1986, Cate and colleagues[9] cloned the bovine and human AMH gene. The human AMH gene is 2.75 kbp in size, has a guanine-cytosine content of approximately 70% and contains 5 exons. The biological activity of the protein is encoded by the fifth and last exon of the gene.[10] The location of the AMH gene is different between species. The AMH gene is located on chromosome 19 in humans[14] and on chromosome 7 in cattle[15] and horses (National Center for Biotechnology Information: gene ID 102148318). Mutations in the AMH gene can result in persistent Müllerian duct syndrome (PMDS), an autosomal-recessive condition in males in which the Müllerian ducts fail to regress.[16] However, not all patients with PMDS have a mutation in the AMH gene; this condition can also arise from a mutation in the AMH receptor gene. Differentiating a mutation in the gene or gene receptor can be accomplished by measuring circulating AMH concentrations. Patients with mutations in receptor gene are characterized by normal circulating AMH concentrations, whereas patients with mutations in the AMH gene usually have undetectable AMH concentrations. Although the majority of the patients with PMDS have mutations in either the AMH gene or receptor, a small percentage of patients (15%) have another underlying cause that has not yet been identified.[17] The relationship between AMH and its receptor to PMDS in the horse has yet to be established.

BIOLOGICAL FUNCTIONS OF ANTI-MÜLLERIAN HORMONE
Sexual Differentiation: Regression of the Müllerian Ducts

Without any doubt, the most important biological function of AMH is to induce regression of the Müllerian ducts in the male fetus. Before sexual differentiation, a fetus contains an undifferentiated gonad along with a pair of Wolffian and Müllerian ducts. In the presence of the SRY gene, the undifferentiated gonad develops into a testis, which produces AMH and testosterone.[18] The production of AMH by the fetal Sertoli cells is of crucial importance in sexual differentiation; the interaction of AMH with the AMH receptor type II induces a cascade of events that result in the regression of the Müllerian ducts.[19] Meanwhile, the production of testosterone by the fetal Leydig cells causes the Wolffian ducts to differentiate into the epididymis, vas deferens, and seminal vesicles. In the absence of the SRY gene, the undifferentiated gonad develops into a fetal ovary.[18] In contrast with the testis, the fetal ovary does not produce AMH or testosterone. As a result, the Müllerian ducts develop into the fallopian tube, uterus, cervix, and cranial end of the vagina and the Wolffian ducts regress. Because the duration of gestation varies between species, there are differences in the period during gestation when the regression of the Müllerian ducts is initiated and completed. The regression of the Müllerian ducts is completed by gestational day 46 in dogs[20] and by day 64 in humans.[21] To date, it is unknown when regression of the Müllerian ducts is initiated or completed in the equine male fetus.

Inhibition of Leydig Cell Differentiation

Although regression of the Müllerian ducts during fetal development is the most important function of AMH, the secretion of AMH in the circulation of males continues after birth until puberty.[22] These relative high circulating AMH concentrations before puberty suggest that AMH also has an important role in males during the postnatal period. As a matter of fact, Behringer and colleagues[23] provided the first evidence that AMH has an influence on Leydig cell differentiation; testicular tissue in AMH deficient mice is characterized by Leydig cell hyperplasia. Moreover, AMH acting through the AMH receptor on the Leydig cells does not only inhibit the differentiation of Leydig cells, but also decreases the steroidogenic activity of Leydig cells. In fact, AMH seems to have a downregulatory effect on the messenger RNA expression of cytochrome P450 17α-hydroxylase/C17 to 20 lyase in Leydig cells.[24] In support of this finding, Rouiller-Fabre and associates[25] demonstrated that testicular steroidogenesis is inhibited by AMH. Based on these studies, it seems that the relatively high concentrations of AMH have a downregulatory role on differentiation and steroidogenic activity of Leydig cells, which might suggest that the quiescent state of the testis before pubertal development is maintained by AMH.

Folliculogenesis

AMH also seems to have an important role in females after birth. Through the use of AMH knockout mice, it became clear that AMH is actively involved in folliculogenesis.[26] Initially, it was shown that the follicular pool is depleted earlier in AMH knockout mice than in wild-type mice. This rapid decline in primordial follicles in AMH knockout mice was attributed to an increased rate of follicular recruitment. Based on these results, it was concluded that the recruitment of primordial follicles is inhibited by AMH.[26,27] The negative influence of AMH on the recruitment of primordial follicles was also examined by assessing follicular growth in the ovary of newborn mice after ovaries were cultured in vitro with or without AMH. Indeed, the number of growing follicles was significantly lower in ovaries cultured with AMH than without AMH.[28] Furthermore, as the number of growing follicles was increased in AMH knockout mice, the possibility exists that the growth of follicle-stimulating hormone (FSH)-sensitive follicles was also reduced by AMH.[26,27] A subsequent study clearly showed that the growth of FSH-sensitive preantral follicles in mice is inhibited by AMH.[29] Likewise, Pellatt and colleagues[30] showed that granulosa cells of growing follicles become less sensitive to FSH in the presence of AMH.

CLINICAL APPLICATIONS OF ANTI-MÜLLERIAN HORMONE IN STALLIONS
Biomarker for Equine Cryptorchidism

Cryptorchidism is a condition in which 1 or both testes are retained within the inguinal canal and/or abdominal cavity. Cryptorchid horses without a scrotal testis are usually presented as geldings with the complaint of displaying stallionlike behavior. Transrectal[31] and transcutaneous (inguinal and abdominal)[32] ultrasound imaging are valuable methods to detect and localize retained testicular tissue. Nonetheless, equine field practitioners routinely use an endocrine test to diagnose cryptorchidism in horses without a scrotal testis because it requires less experience and time compared with ultrasonography. For more than 3 decades, peripheral testosterone and estrogen concentrations have been used by veterinary practitioners as endocrine markers for equine cryptorchidism.[33,34] A recent study showed that AMH can also be used as biomarker for equine cryptorchidism because circulating AMH concentrations are significantly higher in cryptorchid and intact stallions than in geldings. More precisely, circulating AMH concentrations in geldings are either undetectable or approach the lower detection limit of the AMH assay whereas cryptorchid stallions without a descended testis have significantly higher AMH concentrations than intact stallions (**Fig. 2**).[35] This is in contrast to testosterone[36] and estrone sulfate concentrations,[37] which are either significantly lower or not different between cryptorchid stallions and intact stallions. Furthermore, cryptorchid stallions without a descended testis tend to have higher AMH concentrations than cryptorchid stallions with a descended testis, whereas no differences in AMH concentrations were observed between cryptorchid stallions with a descended testis and intact stallions (see **Fig. 2**).[35] Differences in circulating AMH concentrations between cryptorchid stallions without a scrotal testis and intact stallions could be the result of a variety of factors. In human males, the formation of the blood testis barrier at puberty seems to be associated with a decrease in circulating AMH concentrations owing to a redirection in the secretion of AMH from the peripheral circulation into seminal plasma.[22] Considering that a cryptorchid equine testis largely resembles a prepubertal testis,[38] it is plausible that the

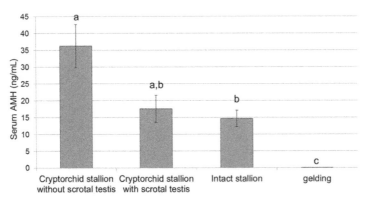

Fig. 2. Circulating anti-Müllerian hormone (AMH) concentrations in cryptorchid stallions with and without a scrotal testis, intact stallions and geldings. Data are presented as mean values ± standard error of the mean. Different letters indicate significant statistical significance (*P*<.05). (*Adapted from* Claes A, Ball BA, Almeida J, et al. Serum anti-Müllerian hormone concentrations in stallions: Developmental changes, seasonal variation, and differences between intact stallions, cryptorchid stallions, and geldings. Theriogenology 2013;79(9):1232–33; with permission from Elsevier.)

secretion of AMH in cryptorchid stallions persists into the peripheral circulation instead of being redirected into the seminal plasma. Second, increasing concentrations of testosterone[39] as well as initiation of meiosis within the seminiferous tubules[40] during pubertal development concurs with a decrease in AMH expression and circulating AMH concentrations in other species. Therefore, arrested spermatogenesis and a reduced expression of androgen receptors[38] in the equine cryptorchid testis could contribute to the higher AMH concentrations observed in cryptorchid stallions compared with intact stallions. Nevertheless, more research is required to elucidate further the mechanism behind the higher AMH concentrations in cryptorchid stallions.

The diagnostic value of AMH to distinguish between geldings and cryptorchid stallions depends on the sensitivity and specificity of the AMH assay to detect retained testicular tissue. Even though this remains to be determined, some data suggest that AMH is more suitable to detect retained testicular tissue than testosterone or estrone sulfate. The specificity of AMH in distinguishing cryptorchid stallions from geldings might be higher than specificity of testosterone[41] because the Sertoli cells of the testis are the only source of AMH in male species, whereas testosterone can be either of testicular or, to a lesser extent, of adrenal origin.[42,43] This could explain the 11% to 14% of inconclusive test results when baseline testosterone concentration was solely used to diagnose cryptorchidism.[36,44] The usefulness of AMH in diagnosing equine cryptorchidism when baseline testosterone concentration failed to do so was also demonstrated in a small number of challenging cases.[41] Despite the low or inconclusive concentration of testosterone, horses with retained testicular tissue could easily be distinguished from geldings, and vice versa, by determining the concentration of AMH in a single blood sample. The results of the AMH assay were confirmed either by an extended human chorionic gonadotropin (hCG) stimulation test in which samples were collected 1 and 24 hours after administration of hCG to detect the biphasic response in testosterone concentrations or by ultrasonography or cryptorchidectomy.[41] Although these preliminary results are promising, more cases are required to confirm this diagnostic advantage of AMH over testosterone.

Among all biomarkers, AMH might be the only endocrine marker that is applicable in all ages. The reliability of baseline or hCG-induced testosterone in identifying cryptorchid stallions is limited in horses younger than 18 months of age[45] and the accuracy of estrone sulfate in detecting retained testicular tissue is considerably reduced in horses before 3 years of age.[44] In contrast, circulating AMH concentrations are high in neonates and prepubertal colts, and even though a decrease in AMH concentrations is observed during puberty, concentrations of AMH remain high in postpubertal stallions.[35] The ability of AMH to detect cryptorchid males during the prepubertal and peripubertal period is clearly demonstrated in cattle[46] and humans.[47] Measuring circulating AMH concentrations is more useful in detecting unilateral cryptorchid calves than baseline or hCG-stimulated testosterone concentrations.[46] In accordance, measurable concentrations of AMH in newborn humans without scrotal testes are indicative of retained testicular tissue.[48] Thus, AMH seems to be the biomarker of choice to detect retained testicular tissue in horses younger than 18 months of age.

As for any other diagnostic markers, it is imperative to be aware of factors that could influence circulating AMH concentrations. First, season has a significant impact on serum AMH concentrations in intact stallions with higher AMH concentrations during the breeding season than during the nonbreeding season.[35] However, it is unclear whether those seasonal variations in AMH concentrations in intact stallions can be extrapolated to cryptorchid stallions. In comparison with testosterone, AMH concentrations are less subjected to diurnal variations as the biological half-life of AMH ($t_{1/2}$ = 1.5 days)[35] is considerably longer than the biological half-life of testosterone ($t_{1/2}$ = 1.1 hour; unpublished data from Dr A. Esteller-Vico, 2014). In conjunction, circulating AMH concentrations decrease rather slow after castration,[35] which is also attributed to the relatively long biological half-life of AMH. Depending on the concentration of AMH before castration, it might take several days to a week before AMH concentrations are reached that are consistent with concentrations in geldings. Therefore, measurement of serum testosterone concentrations might be a better approach than measuring AMH concentrations if testing is warranted in the immediate period (24–48 hours) after castration to confirm that all retained testicular tissue is removed, such as after a questionable cryptorchidectomy. To conclude, AMH has some additional value in the endocrine diagnosis of equine cryptorchidism and, therefore, should be included in the diagnostic workup of cryptorchid horses because it could increase the likelihood of detecting retained testicular tissue, particularly in difficult cases.

Immunohistochemical Biomarker for a Sertoli Cell Tumor

Testicular neoplasia is a rare condition in stallions, which is usually characterized by unilateral or bilateral testicular enlargement.[49] Nonetheless, histopathology is generally required to distinguish between the different types of equine testicular tumors. In humans, it is well-established that AMH can be used to differentiate between Sertoli cell tumors and other types of tumors because AMH is expressed exclusively in sexcord stromal tumors.[50] The immunoexpression of AMH has also been examined in testicular tumors of stallions including Sertoli cell tumors, seminomas and teratomas. Among all examined tumor types, AMH immunolabeling is only present in equine Sertoli cell tumors and localized either to only a small number of neoplastic cells or, to a moderate extent, to the tubular component of the equine Sertoli cell tumor (**Fig. 3**).[51] Despite the heterogeneous expression of AMH in Sertoli cell tumors in different species, detectable AMH immunolabeling is indicative of a Sertoli cell tumor or a mixed tumor containing a Sertoli cell tumor component.[50,51] Along with being an immunohistochemical biomarker, AMH can also serve as a serologic biomarker for Sertoli cell tumors in dogs; dogs with a Sertoli cell tumor had significantly higher circulating AMH concentrations than healthy dogs with no palpable testicular enlargement.[52] Nonetheless, whether the same is true in stallions remains to be determined.

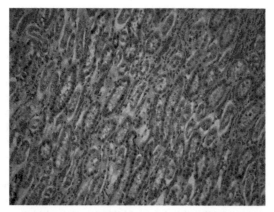

Fig. 3. The immunoexpression of anti-Müllerian hormone (AMH) in an equine Sertoli cell tumor. AMH labeling is localized to the tubular component of the Sertoli cell tumor (H&E).

CLINICAL APPLICATIONS OF ANTI-MÜLLERIAN HORMONE IN MARES
Biomarker for Ovarian Tissue

Besides being synthesized by the Sertoli cells, AMH can also originate from the granulosa cells of the ovarian follicles.[53] Because AMH is an ovarian-specific protein, peripheral AMH concentrations can be used to differentiate between ovariectomized and intact females.[54] In contrast with intact mares, circulating AMH concentrations are undetectable in ovariectomized mares.[55] Nonetheless, undetectable AMH concentrations in mares must be interpreted with some caution in the absence of transrectal examination findings because undetectable AMH concentrations have also been observed in intact older mares with a low number of antral follicles.[56] Notwithstanding this shortcoming, the usefulness of this application in mares is limited at best. In contrast, detection of ovarian tissue is of great importance in small animals especially in case of ovarian remnant syndrome. Intact dogs can be differentiated from spayed dogs using peripheral AMH concentrations with a sensitivity and specificity of approximately 94%. However, the sensitivity of AMH to detect ovarian tissue in dogs is influenced by either pubertal status or age, because it decreases to 50% during the first 6 months of life.[54] Although AMH has some value in differentiating intact from ovariectomized mares, AMH is more widely used in small animals suspected of ovarian remnant syndrome.

Biomarker for Ovarian Reserve and Function

As reported, the ovarian granulosa cells are the only source of AMH in females.[53] The expression of AMH is confined to the cytoplasm of equine granulosa cells and changes during follicular development (**Fig. 4**). The primary follicle is the first type of ovarian follicle displaying AMH expression and as the number of granulosa cells layers increases so does the expression of AMH.[57] Moreover, the expression of AMH is strong in small antral follicles (15–20 mm) but decreases around follicle selection resulting in only faint AMH labeling in dominant and preovulatory follicles.[58] In addition to follicle type, follicular viability is another factor that has an influence on the expression of AMH in equine ovarian follicles. As opposed to viable follicles, only weak AMH expression is detected in granulosa cells of atretic follicles.[57] Thus, the expression of AMH in equine granulosa cells is influenced by follicular development and viability.

Considering that AMH is synthesized exclusively by the ovarian follicles, it seems likely that circulating AMH concentrations are a reflection of the size of the follicular pool. Indeed, a strong mutual relationship exists between circulating AMH concentrations, antral follicle count (AFC) and the number of primordial follicles in women and mice.[59,60] Consequently, circulating AMH concentrations as well as AFC are commonly used to assess ovarian reserve in women. In addition, the onset of menopause in women can be predicted reasonably well using circulating AMH concentrations.[61] In contrast with women, aged mares do not go through menopause but can experience ovarian senescence, a condition somewhat similar to menopause. Early signs of ovarian senescence are prolonged interovulatory intervals, smaller preovulatory follicles, and a low number of antral follicles. Eventually, the follicular pool becomes depleted, resulting in ovulation failure and cessation of estrous cycles.[62] As in humans, AMH could have some usefulness in assessing the size of the follicular pool in aged mares. In fact, circulating AMH concentrations are correlated positively with AFC in middle-aged and aged mares but not in young mares, and the correlation between AMH and AFC is moderate in middle-aged mares and strong in aged mares. Also, aged mares have significantly lower AMH concentrations and AFC compared with middle-aged mares, indicating that the size of the follicular pool in mares declines

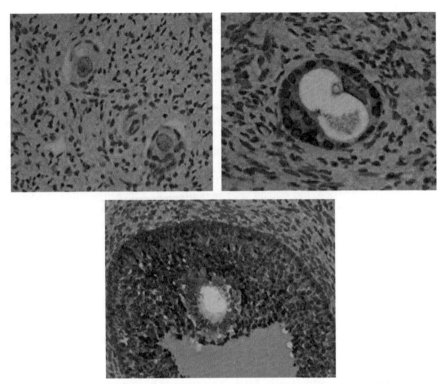

Fig. 4. The expression of anti-Müllerian hormone (AMH) in equine primordial, preantral, and antral follicles (from *left to right*) using immunohistochemistry. No AMH expression is present within primordial follicles, whereas mild expression of AMH can be detected within the granulosa cells of a primary follicle. The expression of AMH increases with follicular development; granulosa cells of antral follicles display stronger AMH labeling (H&E, 200×). (*Adapted from* Ball BA, Conley AJ, MacLaughlin DT, et al. Expression of anti-Müllerian hormone (AMH) in equine granulosa-cell tumors and in normal equine ovaries. Theriogenology 2008;70(6):974; with permission from Elsevier.)

with age. Irrespective of these age-related decreases in AMH and AFC, distinct differences in circulating AMH concentrations and AFC have been observed among young, middle-aged, and aged mares. This, in turn, might indicate that the size of the follicular pool is inherently different between mares of the same age and, therefore, the reproductive age of a mare must be distinguished from the calendar age.[56] Finally, AMH is particularly suitable as biomarker for ovarian reserve in mares because concentrations of AMH are relatively stable during and between different estrous cycles,[56] and this stability is likely owing to the long biological half-life of AMH (1.9 days).[55] Thus, AMH seems to be a reflection of population of follicles in mares and could be valuable in assessing the reproductive life-span of aged mares.

More in-depth research suggests that variations in circulating AMH concentrations are also a reflection of follicular function. Distinct molecular differences have been detected between granulosa cells of growing follicles of mares with high and low AMH concentrations. Low circulating AMH concentrations are associated with a low expression of AMH, AMH receptor type 2, estrogen receptor 1, estrogen receptor 2, inhibin alpha, and follitropin receptor in granulosa cells of growing follicles.[58] It is well-established that these genes play a crucial role in folliculogenesis and a reduced expression in other species seems to be linked to reduced oocyte quality,[63] responsiveness to FSH,[64] and granulosa cell proliferation.

Biomarker for Equine Granulosa Cell Tumors

The equine granulosa cell tumor (GCT), a sex-cord stromal tumor, is the most common tumor of the equine ovary. Although rarely metastatic, equine GCTs are usually associated with changes in behavior such as failure to cycle, stallionlike behavior, or persistent estrus (nymphomania). Other diagnostic features of a classical GCT in mares are a unilaterally enlarged ovary with a honeycomb appearance on ultrasonography and a contralateral inactive ovary. Similar findings can occasionally be observed in mares with a hemorrhagic anovulatory follicle or ovarian hematoma but, in contrast with those ovarian conditions, the equine GCT is hormonally active. Therefore, a crucial step in the diagnostic workup of a mare with a GCT is an endocrine analysis, which includes the measurement of progesterone, testosterone, and inhibin. Low progesterone concentrations in conjunction with increased concentrations of inhibin and/or testosterone are indicative of a GCT. Inhibin concentrations are increased in nearly 90% of GCT mares and testosterone concentrations are increased in approximately 50% to 60% of the GCT cases.[65] Nonetheless, concentrations of testosterone[66] and inhibin[67] are also increased during pregnancy, whereas slightly increased testosterone concentrations in nonpregnant mares could be attributed to increased adrenal gland activity.[42] In contrast, a small percentage of mares with a GCT do not have increased concentrations of inhibin or testosterone. In such cases, it can be challenging to diagnose a GCT using the conventional endocrine markers, namely, inhibin and testosterone.

Besides inhibin and testosterone, AMH also proves to be important in the diagnosis of equine GCTs.[55,57,68] AMH is heterogeneously expressed in equine GCTs and present in sera of GCT mares in a bioactive form because it is able to induce regression of the Müllerian ducts in an in vitro assay.[57] More important, at least clinically, mares with a GCT have higher circulating AMH concentrations than nonpregnant and pregnant mares without a GCT indicating that AMH can serve as an endocrine marker for equine GCTs. Interestingly, AMH turns out to be the most important endocrine marker to identify mares with a GCT because it has a higher sensitivity (98%) than testosterone (48%), inhibin (80%), or testosterone and inhibin combined (84%).[68] Another important of advantage is that AMH can be used to detect GCTs in pregnant mares because circulating AMH concentrations are not influenced by gestation,[55] whereas testosterone[66] and inhibin[67] concentrations are increased during gestation. Furthermore, circulating AMH concentrations in nonpregnant mares are more stable throughout the cycle[55] than testosterone or inhibin concentrations, which are influenced by the stage of the cycle.[69,70] Finally, data in other species indicate that AMH has an inhibitory effect on the growth of antral follicles.[68] Hence, AMH might be involved in suppressing follicular development on the contralateral inactive ovary but more research is required to confirm this hypothesis.[57] To conclude, it is apparent that AMH is not only more widely applicable but also improves the diagnostic accuracy of the current equine GCT panel.

REFERENCES

1. Jost A. Recherches sur la differentiation sexuelle de l'embryon de lapin. III. role des gonades foetales dans la differenciation sexuelle somatique. Arch Anat Microsc Morphol Exp 1947;36:271–315.

2. Jost A. Problems of fetal endocrinology: the gonadal and hypophyseal hormones. Recent Prog Horm Res 1953;8:379–418.

3. Josso N, Cate RL, Picard JY, et al. Anti-Mullerian hormone: the Jost factor. Recent Prog Horm Res 1993;48:1–59.

4. Josso N. Permeability of membranes to the Müllerian-inhibiting substance synthesized by the human fetal testis in vitro: a clue to its biochemical nature. J Clin Endocrinol Metab 1972;34(2):265–70.

5. Budzik GP, Swann DA, Hayashi A, et al. Enhanced purification of Mullerian inhibiting substance by lectin affinity-chromatography. Cell 1980;21(3):909–15.

6. Picard JY, Tran D, Josso N. Biosynthesis of labeled anti-Mullerian hormone by fetal testes - evidence for glycoprotein nature of hormone and for its disulfide-bonded structure. Mol Cell Endocrinol 1978;12(1):17–30.

7. Picard JY, Josso N. Purification of testicular anti-Mullerian hormone allowing direct visualization of the pure glycoprotein and determination of yield and purification factor. Mol Cell Endocrinol 1984;34(1):23–9.

8. Picard JY, Goulut C, Bourrillon R, et al. Biochemical-analysis of bovine testicular anti-Mullerian hormone. FEBS Lett 1986;195(1–2):73–6.

9. Cate RL, Mattaliano RJ, Hession C, et al. Isolation of the bovine and human genes for Mullerian inhibiting substance and expression of the human gene in animal cells. Cell 1986;45(5):685–98.

10. Josso N, Clemente N. Transduction pathway of anti-Mullerian hormone, a sex-specific member of the TGF-beta family. Trends Endocrinol Metab 2003;14(2):91–7.

11. Pepinsky RB, Sinclair LK, Chow EP, et al. Proteolytic processing of Mullerian inhibiting substance produces a transforming growth factor-beta-like fragment. J Biol Chem 1988;263(35):18961–4.

12. MacLaughlin DT, Hudson PL, Graciano AL, et al. Mullerian duct regression and antiproliferative bioactivities of Mullerian inhibiting substance reside in its carboxy-terminal domain. Endocrinology 1992;131(1):291–6.

13. Wilson CA, di Clemente N, Ehrenfels C, et al. Mullerian inhibiting substance requires its N-terminal domain for maintenance of biological activity, a novel finding within the transforming growth factor-beta superfamily. Mol Endocrinol 1993;7(2):247–57.

14. Cohen-Haguenauer O, Picard JY, Mattei MG, et al. Mapping of the gene for anti-Mullerian hormone to the short arm of human chromosome 19. Cytogenet Cell Genet 1987;44(1):2–6.

15. Gao Q, Womack JE. A genetic map of bovine chromosome 7 with an interspecific hybrid backcross panel. Mamm Genome 1997;8(4):258–61.

16. Knebelmann B, Boussin L, Guerrier D, et al. Anti-Mullerian hormone Bruxelles: a nonsense mutation associated with the persistent Mullerian duct syndrome. Proc Natl Acad Sci U S A 1991;88(9):3767–71.

17. Josso N, Belville C, di Clemente N, et al. AMH and AMH receptor defects in persistent Mullerian duct syndrome. Hum Reprod Update 2005;11(4):351–6.

18. Nef S, Parada LF. Hormones in male sexual development. Genes Dev 2000;14(24):3075–86.

19. Jenny AV. AMH signaling: from receptor to target gene. Mol Cell Endocrinol 2003;211(1–2):65–73.

20. Meyerswallen VN, Manganaro TF, Kuroda T, et al. The critical period for Mullerian duct regression in the dog embryo. Biol Reprod 1991;45(4):626–33.

21. Taguchi O, Cunha GR, Lawrence WD, et al. Timing and irreversibility of Mullerian duct inhibition in the embryonic reproductive tract of the human male. Dev Biol 1984;106(2):394–8.

22. Rey R, Lukas-Croisier C, Lasala C, et al. AMH/MIS: what we know already about the gene, the protein and its regulation. Mol Cell Endocrinol 2003;211(1–2): 21–31.

23. Behringer RR, Finegold MJ, Cate RL. Mullerian-inhibiting substance function during mammalian sexual development. Cell 1994;79(3):415–25.

24. Racine C, Rey R, Forest MG, et al. Receptors for anti-Mullerian hormone on Leydig cells are responsible for its effects on steroidogenesis and cell differentiation. Proc Natl Acad Sci U S A 1998;95(2):594–9.

25. Rouiller-Fabre V, Carmona S, Merhi RA, et al. Effect of anti-Mullerian hormone on Sertoli and Leydig cell functions in fetal and immature rats. Endocrinology 1998; 139(3):1213–20.

26. Durlinger ALL, Kramer P, Karels B, et al. Control of primordial follicle recruitment by anti-Mullerian hormone in the mouse ovary. Endocrinology 1999;140(12): 5789–96.

27. Durlinger ALL, Visser JA, Themmen APN. Regulation of ovarian function: the role of anti-Mullerian hormone. Reproduction 2002;124(5):601–9.

28. Durlinger AL, Gruijters MJ, Kramer P, et al. Anti-Mullerian hormone inhibits initiation of primordial follicle growth in the mouse ovary. Endocrinology 2002;143(3): 1076–84.

29. Durlinger ALL, Gruijters MJG, Kramer P, et al. Anti-Mullerian hormone attenuates the effects of FSH on follicle development in the mouse ovary. Endocrinology 2001;142(11):4891–9.

30. Pellatt L, Rice S, Dilaver N, et al. Anti-Mullerian hormone reduces follicle sensitivity to follicle-stimulating hormone in human granulosa cells. Fertil Steril 2011; 96(5):1246–51.

31. Jann HW, Rains JR. Diagnostic ultrasonography for evaluation of cryptorchidism in horses. J Am Vet Med Assoc 1990;196(2):297–300.

32. Schambourg MA, Farley JA, Marcoux M, et al. Use of transabdominal ultrasonography to determine the location of cryptorchid testes in the horse. Equine Vet J 2006;38(3):242–5.

33. Cox JE, Williams JH, Rowe PH, et al. Testosterone in normal, cryptorchid and castrated male horses. Equine Vet J 1973;5(2):85–90.

34. Ganjam VK. An inexpensive, yet precise, laboratory diagnostic method to confirm cryptorchidism in horse. Proceedings of the Annual Convention of the American Association of Equine Practitioners Vancouver (BC) 1977;23:245–50.

35. Claes A, Ball BA, Almeida J, et al. Serum anti-Mullerian hormone concentrations in stallions: developmental changes, seasonal variation, and differences between intact stallions, cryptorchid stallions, and geldings. Theriogenology 2013;79(9): 1229–35.

36. Arighi M, Bosu WTK. Comparison of hormonal methods for diagnosis of cryptorchidism in horses. J Equine Vet Sci 1989;9(1):20–6.

37. Carneiro GF, Liu IKM, Illera JC, et al. Enzyme immunoassay for the measurement of estrone sulphate in cryptorchids, stallions and donkeys. Proceedings of the Annual Convention of the American Association of Equine Practitioners, Baltimore (MD) 1998;44:3–4.

38. Almeida J, Conley AJ, Ball BA. Expression of anti-Müllerian hormone, CDKN1B, connexin 43, androgen receptor and steroidogenic enzymes in the equine cryptorchid testis. Equine Vet J 2013;45(5):538–45.

39. Rey R, Lordereau-Richard I, Carel JC, et al. Anti-Mullerian hormone and testosterone serum levels are inversely during normal and precocious pubertal development. J Clin Endocrinol Metab 1993;77(5):1220–6.

40. Al-Attar L, Noel K, Dutertre M, et al. Hormonal and cellular regulation of Sertoli cell anti-Mullerian hormone production in the postnatal mouse. J Clin Invest 1997; 100(6):1335–43.

41. Claes A, Ball BA, Corbin CJ, et al. Anti-Müllerian hormone as a diagnostic marker for equine cryptorchidism in three cases with equivocal testosterone concentrations. J Equine Vet Sci 2014;34(0):442–5.

42. Morganti M, Conley AJ, Vico AE, et al. Stallion-like behavior in mares: What is the role of the adrenal glands? Proceedings of the Annual Convention of the American Association of Equine Practitioners, Baltimore (MD) 2010;56:314.

43. Silberzahn P, Rashed F, Zwain I, et al. Androstenedione and testosterone biosynthesis by the adrenal cortex of the horse. Steroids 1984;43(2):147–52.

44. Cox JE, Redhead PH, Dawson FE. Comparison of the measurement of plasma testosterone and plasma estrogens for the diagnosis of cryptorchidism in the horse. Equine Vet J 1986;18(3):179–82.

45. Cox JE. Experiences with a diagnostic test for equine cryptorchidism. Equine Vet J 1975;7(4):179–83.

46. Kitahara G, El-Sheikh Ali H, Sato T, et al. Anti-Mullerian hormone (AMH) profiles as a novel biomarker to evaluate the existence of a functional cryptorchid testis in Japanese black calves. J Reprod Dev 2012;58(3):310–5.

47. Lee MM, Donahoe PK, Silverman BL, et al. Measurements of serum Mullerian inhibiting substance in the evaluation of children with nonpalpable gonads. N Engl J Med 1997;336(21):1480–6.

48. Guibourdenche J, Lucidarme N, Chevenne D, et al. Anti-Mullerian hormone levels in serum from human foetuses and children: pattern and clinical interest. Mol Cell Endocrinol 2003;211(1–2):55–63.

49. Brinsko SP. Neoplasia of the male reproductive tract. Vet Clin North Am Equine Pract 1998;14(3):517–33.

50. Rey R, Sabourin JC, Venara M, et al. Anti-Mullerian hormone is a specific marker of Sertoli- and granulosa-cell origin in gonadal tumors. Hum Pathol 2000;31(10): 1202–8.

51. Ball BA, Conley AJ, Grundy SA, et al. Expression of anti-Mullerian hormone (AMH) in the equine testis. Theriogenology 2008;69(5):624–31.

52. Holst BS, Dreimanis U. Anti-Mullerian hormone: a potentially useful biomarker for the diagnosis of canine Sertoli cell tumours. BMC Vet Res 2015;11:166.

53. Rajpert-De Meyts E, Jorgensen N, Graem N, et al. Expression of anti-Mullerian hormone during normal and pathological gonadal development: association with differentiation of Sertoli and granulosa cells. J Clin Endocrinol Metab 1999; 84(10):3836–44.

54. Place NJ, Hansen BS, Cheraskin JL, et al. Measurement of serum anti-Mullerian hormone concentration in female dogs and cats before and after ovariohysterectomy. J Vet Diagn Invest 2011;23(3):524–7.

55. Almeida J, Ball BA, Conley AJ, et al. Biological and clinical significance of anti-Mullerian hormone determination in blood serum of the mare. Theriogenology 2011;76(8):1393–403.

56. Claes A, Ball BA, Scoggin KE, et al. The interrelationship between anti-Müllerian hormone, ovarian follicular populations, and age in mares. Equine Vet J 2015; 47(5):537–41.

57. Ball BA, Conley AJ, MacLaughlin DT, et al. Expression of anti-Mullerian hormone (AMH) in equine granulosa-cell tumors and in normal equine ovaries. Theriogenology 2008;70(6):968–77.

58. Claes A, Ball BA, Troedsson MH, et al. Molecular changes in the equine follicle in relation to variations in antral follicle count and anti-Mullerian hormone concentrations. Equine Vet J 2015. http://dx.doi.org/10.1111/evj.12514.

59. Hansen KR, Hodnett GM, Knowlton N, et al. Correlation of ovarian reserve tests with histologically determined primordial follicle number. Fertil Steril 2011;95(1): 170–5.

60. Kevenaar ME, Meerasahib MF, Kramer P, et al. Serum anti-Mullerian hormone levels reflect the size of the primordial follicle pool in mice. Endocrinology 2006;147(7):3228–34.

61. Tehrani FR, Shakeri N, Solaymani-Dodaran M, et al. Predicting age at menopause from serum antiMullerian hormone concentration. Menopause 2011;18(7): 766–70.

62. Carnevale EM, Bergfelt DR, Ginther OJ. Follicular activity and concentrations of FSH and LH associated with senescence in mares. Anim Reprod Sci 1994; 35(3-4):231–46.

63. Ireland JJ, Zielak-Steciwko AE, Jimenez-Krassel F, et al. Variation in the ovarian reserve is linked to alterations in intrafollicular estradiol production and ovarian biomarkers of follicular differentiation and oocyte quality in cattle. Biol Reprod 2009;80(5):954–64.

64. Scheetz D, Folger JK, Smith GW, et al. Granulosa cells are refractory to FSH action in individuals with a low antral follicle count. Reprod Fertil Dev 2011;24(2): 327–36.

65. McCue PM, Roser JF, Munro CJ, et al. Granulosa cell tumors of the equine ovary. Vet Clin North Am Equine Pract 2006;22(3):799–817.

66. Silberzahn P, Zwain I, Martin B. Concentration increase of unbound testosterone in plasma of the mare throughout pregnancy. Endocrinology 1984;115(1):416–9.

67. Nambo Y, Nagata S, Oikawa M, et al. High concentrations of immunoreactive inhibin in the plasma of mares and fetal gonads during the second half of pregnancy. Reprod Fertil Dev 1996;8(8):1137–45.

68. Ball BA, Almeida J, Conley AJ. Determination of serum anti-Mullerian hormone concentrations for the diagnosis of granulosa-cell tumours in mares. Equine Vet J 2013;45(2):199–203.

69. Roser JF, McCue PM, Hoye E. Inhibin activity in the mare and stallion. Domest Anim Endocrinol 1994;11(1):87–100.

70. Bergfelt DR, Mann BG, Schwartz NB, et al. Circulating concentrations of immuno-reactive inhibin and FSH during the estrous cycle of mares. J Equine Vet Sci 1991;11(6):319–22.

Endometritis

Managing Persistent Post-Breeding Endometritis

Igor F. Canisso, DVM, MSc, PhD[a], Jamie Stewart, DVM, MS[a],
Marco A. Coutinho da Silva, DVM, MSc, PhD[b],*

KEYWORDS

- Mare • Endometritis • Post-Breeding endometritis • Uterine lavage
- Intrauterine fluid

KEY POINTS

- Susceptible mares have impaired uterine defense mechanisms.
- Persistent post-breeding induced endometritis is characterized by abnormal imbalance in pro-inflammatory and anti-inflammatory cytokines.
- Diagnosis can be made through endometrial histology, culture, cytology, and/or ultrasound; each of which have differing advantages and disadvantages.
- The most common management strategies include combinations of therapeutic techniques such as uterine lavage and ecbolic treatments that enhance drainage of the persistent uterine fluid.

INTRODUCTION

Mares have been classified as susceptible and resistant to endometritis based on their ability to clear bacteria from the reproductive tract following experimental inoculation through the cervix.[1–6] Clinically, mares are classified as susceptible to endometritis based on the persistent presence of intra-uterine fluid accumulation by 24 to 48 hours post-breeding.[7] For years, it was thought that post-breeding endometritis was solely caused by infectious agents, particularly bacteria.[5,8] However, a seminal study demonstrated that estrous mares infused with either bacteria (*Streptococcus zooepidemicus*) or spermatozoa presented similar number of neutrophils in the uterine fluid at 4 hours post uterine infusion.[9] The results of this study established the concept that post-breeding endometritis is a normal physiologic, transient inflammatory response

[a] Department of Veterinary Clinical Medicine, College of Veterinary Medicine, University of Illinois Urbana-Champaign, 2001 S Lincoln Ave, Urbana, IL 61822, USA; [b] Department of Veterinary Clinical Sciences, College of Veterinary Medicine, The Ohio State University, 601 Vernon Tharp St, Columbus, OH 43210, USA
* Corresponding author.
E-mail address: marco.dasilva@cvm.osu.edu

that serves the purpose to clear the uterus from excess of sperm cells, seminal plasma, debris and bacterial contaminants.[5,10]

Persistent post-breeding endometritis is a prolonged (ie, longer than 48 h) inflammatory response of the endometrium caused by spermatozoa and is estimated to affect approximately 10% to 15% of mares.[7] In some cases, bacterial contamination may also be present. Therefore, the objectives of this article are to discuss some of the most relevant literature concerning persistent post-breeding endometritis and the authors' clinical experiences managing this condition in ambulatory practice and referring hospitals.

UTERINE DEFENSE MECHANISMS
Reproductive Tract Barriers to Prevent Uterine Infection

Vulva, vestibule-vagina sphincter, and cervix represent three physical barriers or seals in the mare reproductive tract to prevent uterine infections. If one of these barriers is not functional, the mare will be prone to pneumovagina and pneumometra (physometra), causing irritation of the uterus and potential aspiration of bacteria. The vulva, an outward barrier against infection, should have perfectly apposed lips and be vertically oriented withe 2/3 of the vulvar length located below the pelvic brim and 1/3 of the vulvar length above the pelvic brim (**Fig. 1**).

The vestibule-vagina sphincter is the only barrier that remains functional while the mare is in estrus and helps to prevent aspiration of air and debris into the cranial vagina. However, it is also a common site for lacerations during foaling, and its integrity and competency should be assessed during breeding soundness examinations. When performing vaginoscopy, the sphincter should offer some resistance to the passage of the speculum. While advancing or retracting the vaginal speculum, the sphincter should close like curtains in front of the opening of the speculum. Another method consists of physically separating the vulvar lips with hands and fingers as wide as possible, and listening for any noise of air being aspirated into the cranial vagina, which would denote an incompetent vestibule-vagina sphincter. Additionally, if the vestibule-vaginal sphincter is incompetent, the operator may be able to directly visualize the vagina and cervix (**Fig. 2**). The cervix should be free from lacerations and adhesions, relaxed and open during estrus, and be tight and closed during diestrus and pregnancy.

Uterine Immune Response

Following intrauterine deposition of semen, there is initiation of a complement system which is responsible for chemotaxis and activation of polymorphonuclear neutrophils (PMNs) to the uterine lumen as soon as 30 minutes after insemination.[5,11] The activated PMNs then function to remove bacteria, debris, and sperm cells from the uterus through phagocytosis.[3,12] Neutrophil extracellular traps (NETs) (ie, extracellular fibers of DNA) also begin to form and appear to play a major role in the uterine clearance post-breeding by binding to pathogens but not sperm.[13] Rebordão and collaborators[14] found that mares suffering from S zooepidemicus or E. coli endometritis formed NETs in vivo, demonstrating a potential complementary mechanism by which mares can resist endometritis.[14] Further work is still warranted to determine if and how impaired NET formation occurs in mares susceptible to infectious endometritis. While NETs may play a crucial role in preventing bacterial endometritis, they also release inflammatory mediators that some speculate could lead to endometrial degenerative disease.[15] Overstimulation of NET formation and/or a decrease in NET degradation have been postulated as potential causes for increased endometrial fibrosis and

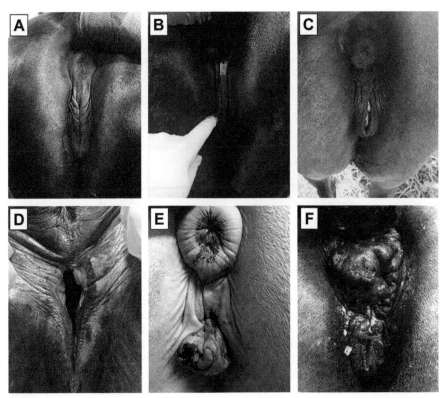

Fig. 1. (*A*) Normal vulvar conformation in a broodmare. Note the vertically oriented vulva, perfect apposition of vulvar lips, and 2/3 of the vulvar length is located below the pelvic brim. (*B*) The maiden mare represented in this picture has a slightly sunken anus, and vulvar 2/3 of the vulvar length is located above the pelvic brim. The vulvar labia on this mare is very weak and has minimal fat pad surrounding the vulva making the mare prone to pneumo-vagina. (*C*) Vulva of an older broodmare, note the recessed anus and imperfect apposition of the vulvar lips; (*D*) Quarter horse mare with torn perineal body; (*E*) Paint Horse vulvar squamous cell carcinoma. (*F*) Older Andalusian mare presenting melanoma in the vulva, note the imperfect apposition of the labia and deformed vulva as a consequence of these masses, this mare is prone to air aspiration. Lindsey Rothrock is acknowledged for taking the picture F to the authors.

subsequent endometrial secretory function impairment,[15] though no data currently exists to support this hypothesis.

After breeding, there is an increase in myometrium contractility likely induced by PGF2α from endometrium and membranes from activated PMNs (ie, via metabolism of arachidonic acidic through cyclooxygenases) that aid in eliminating sperm and fluid through the cervix.[16,17] Mares susceptible to endometritis seem to have an impaired ability to evacuate the uterine fluid after breeding,[18,19] which can be harmful to both sperm and developing embryos.[12] Compromised uterine contractility is mediated by increased endometrial production of nitric oxide, a potent muscle relaxant.[20] Nitric ox-ide was found to be elevated after breeding in mares susceptible to endometritis when compared to resistant mares.[21] While it is clear that nitric oxide plays a role in persis-tent post-breeding endometritis, it is unclear whether it is causative or an effect of the underlying pathogenesis.

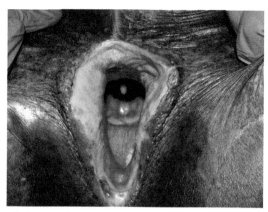

Fig. 2. Evaluation of the vestibule-vagina sphincter in a broodmare. The sphincter was incompetent allowing direct visualization of the cranial vagina.

Cytokines also play a key role in modulating inflammatory response in normal mares and mares susceptible to endometritis. Woodward and collaborators[21] found that at around 6 hours post-insemination, susceptible mares had lower mRNA expressions of the pro-inflammatory cytokine IL6 and the anti-inflammatory cytokines IL10 and IL1RA (IL1RN), which occur in response to pathogens and are needed to resolve inflammation. The same authors also reported that IL1β, a pro-inflammatory cytokine, was found to be increased at both 2 and 6 hours in both susceptible and resistant mares, suggesting a normal mechanism in the initial transient endometritis response. Interferon gamma (IFNγ) expression, important for initiation of the inflammation cascade, was both delayed in onset and slower to return to pre-insemination levels in susceptible mares, consistent with clinical signs of prolonged inflammation and infertility.[21] Cytokine response to inflammation is the first step in recognition and elimination of foreign debris; therefore, an altered local cytokine response, as has been demonstrated in susceptible mares, likely contributes to impaired uterine clearance and subsequent infertility in susceptible mares.[21] (**Fig. 3**)

Recently, studies have also suggested that CRISP-3 (unpublished personal communication M Troedsson) and lactoferrin,[22] two highly abundant seminal plasma proteins, may play a role in protecting viable sperm and opsonizing dead non-viable sperm following breeding. These studies suggest that the seminal plasma may play a role in the modulation of post-breeding uterine inflammation and require further investigation.

DIAGNOSIS

A detailed approach on various diagnostic modalities for endometritis is presented in Ryan A. Ferris's article, "Endometritis: Diagnostic Tools for Infectious Endometritis," in this issue, thus the reader is referred to consult that article for description of the various methods, and thus herein we will provide an overview of the most commonly used diagnostic techniques used as part of the breeding management of mares susceptible to endometritis.

The diagnosis of endometritis in mares is complicated by its multi-factorial nature. As previously mentioned, the different causes can overlap leading to a multitude of problems. Often the diagnosis of persistent post-breeding endometritis is attained after breeding, and prediction of susceptibility is often limited to reproductive history of

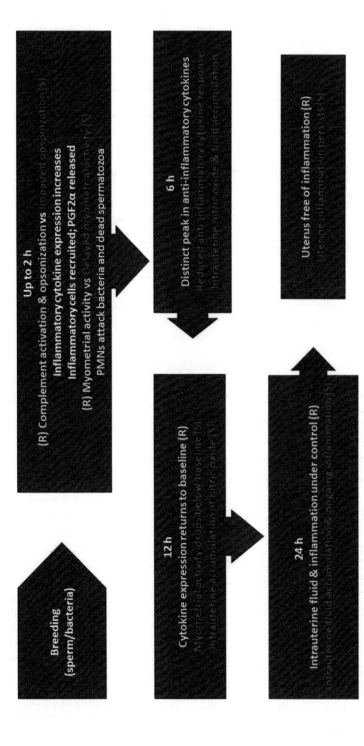

Fig. 3. Suggested sequence of events involved in persistent breeding induced endometritis. (*From* Woodward EM, Troedsson MH. Equine breeding-induced endometritis: a review. J Equine Vet Sci 2013;33(9):673–82; with permission.)

failure to conceive and excessive intrauterine fluid accumulation after breeding.[23] Risk factors for susceptibility (**Table 1**) can be used to estimate whether a mare presented for breeding may be susceptible to endometritis. For example, infectious endometritis may be associated with persistent post-breeding endometritis due to the mare's inability to clear excess fluid and debris post-mating. Being able to identify the underlying pathology can help to determine the best management strategy, which is the subject of many recent publications. Historically, diagnosis and treatment of endometritis has been focused in "problem mares", or those with clinical endometritis. However, recent work has found the rate of apparently healthy mares with subclinical endometritis to be as high as 28.6%, highlighting the importance of pre-breeding examinations in all mares.[24]

Endometrial Sampling: Cytology, Culture and Histopathology

Endometrial cytology is a quick way to diagnose endometrial inflammation in the mare. However, an accurate cytologic interpretation relies on a collection technique that yields a high number of well-preserved cells representative of a large uterine surface area.[25] Endometrial cytology can be performed by guarded cotton swabs, cytobrush, low-volume uterine lavage, or by recovery of intrauterine fluid with an artificial insemination pipette.

A study demonstrated that cytobrush technique combined with culture decreased the likelihood of a false negative result[26]; thus, the use of cytobrush is the preferred technique over cotton swab for routine diagnosis of endometritis.

When evaluating endometrial cytology, a threshold value of $\geq$1% PMN cells per high-power field and/or culture of a single bacterial isolate was associated with reduced live foaling rates. These results exhibited high specificity (0.94), meaning that mares with a negative diagnosis were highly likely to produce live foals, but a very low sensitivity (0.08), meaning that a mare with a positive diagnosis could still produce a live foal, but were less likely to than a mare without clinical signs of endometritis.[27]

Bacterial culture may provide important diagnostic information in cases of infectious endometritis or to rule out non-infectious endometritis, as growth of microorganisms

Table 1 Incidence of risk factors for endometritis in Sport Horses (n = 513 cycles)	
Risk Factors	# of Estrous Cycles (% Incidence)
Abnormal breeding history	51(8)
Positive endometrial culture	40(7)
$\geq$2 cm endometrial fluid prior to breeding	74(12)
Abnormal perineal conformation	89(15)
Abnormal cervix	25(4)
Post-breeding endometrial >1.5 <2 cm	23(4)
Post-breeding fluid $\geq$2 cm	120(20)
Post-foaling vulvo-plasty (Caslick procedure) not repaired after episiotomy	29(5)
Abnormalities of the reproductive tract	46(8)
Post-breeding fluid persistent after 36 h after breeding	72(12)

Adapted from Bucca S, Carli A, Buckley T, et al. The use of dexamethasone administered to mares at breeding time in the modulation of persistent mating induced endometritis. Theriogenology 2008;70:1093–100.

has been associated with reduced pregnancy rates.[2,27] However, as with any diagnostic test, false positives and false negatives may result from poor sampling techniques. One of the most commonly used sampling techniques is a guarded culture swab, which has the advantages of being cheap, easy, and safe to use. However, swabs only come into contact with a 1 to 2 cm area of endometrium, making a false negative result likely.[28] A low-volume uterine flush, is a reasonable alternative sampling technique with an estimated sensitivity and specificity of 0.71 and 0.86, respectively.[28] While more difficult to perform, this technique shows a sensitivity twice as high as those reported for uterine swabs (0.34 and 0.33) by Nielsen[29] and Overbeck and colleagues,[26] respectively. Since this method of cytologic evaluation of the flush efflux is timely and not practical for use by clinicians, Christoffersen and colleagues[30] described a double-guarded flushing technique, which exhibited a comparable sensitivity (0.75) and specificity (0.72) to the previous technique without the need for evaluation of the flush efflux to rule out false-positive samples from contamination. In the authors' practices, we used cytobrush and swab culture for routine screening and reserve small volume uterine lavage culture and cytology for mares with history of subfertility, such as being barren for one or more years and with recurrent embryonic losses.

Endometrial biopsy is expensive and it is not practical for every case, thus in the authors' practices, this technique is used as part of the breeding soundness evaluation of mares and can be used to obtain a sample that will be submitted to aerobic culture, as previously reported.[29] The presence of polymorphonuclear cells in the luminal epithelium and stratum compactum of the endometrium on histology are indicative of inflammation/infection. Kenney & Doig[31] introduced a scoring system in which mares were classified into 4 categories according to the acute and chronic changes observed in the histopathology of the endometrium. Though this classification system can predict the ability of a mare to carry a foal to term, it does not determine the ability of the mare to become pregnant.[32,33] Therefore, the use of uterine biopsies to diagnose cases of post-breeding endometritis is limited.

Ultrasound Examination

In mares with persistent post-breeding endometritis, the major consequence of impaired uterine clearance is increased uterine fluid retention and persistent inflammation or edema of the endometrium, which occurs more frequently in older or barren mares and is associated with reduced fertility.[34] This may be partially due to the build-up of nitric oxide in susceptible mares that could cause myometrial relaxation, leading to decreased clearance of fluids. Intra-uterine fluid accumulation measuring greater than 2 cm in height on transrectal ultrasound during estrus prior to breeding were more likely to be susceptible to persistent breeding induced endometritis (**Fig. 4**).[35] Using an endometrial edema scoring system (0 absent and 4 excessive edema), Rasmussen and colleagues[24] found that the mares with a score of 3 (strong edema), or 4 (excessive edema) early in estrus were 5.48 times more likely to have a positive culture of S zooepidemicus post-breeding than those with a score of 2 (moderate edema). These results confirm the standard clinical practice of checking mares post-breeding not only for ovulation, but to assess the presence and type of fluid post-breeding.

MANAGEMENT STRATEGIES FOR SUSCEPTIBLE MARES

Overall treatment for persistent breeding induced endometritis includes a combination of antimicrobials, correction of anatomic defects and management strategies to control/modulate uterine inflammation.

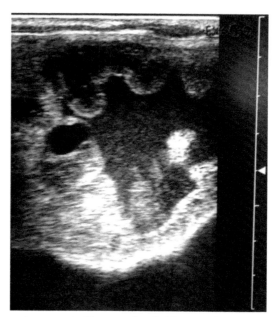

Fig. 4. Large echogenic amount of intrauterine fluid accumulation in an older broodmare post-breeding.

Antimicobials

Antimicrobials may be used in treatment and or prevention of post-breeding induced endometritis.[36] Post-breeding intra-uterine infusion of antimicrobials is a standard method used to prevent uterine infection mainly in Thoroughbreds mares. However, there is no evidence-based data supporting that this practice actually improves conception rates or prevent infection. It is likely that a single antibiotic infusion post-breeding will not prevent bacterial infection.[36]

The use of repeated intrauterine infusions of antibiotics may also lead to disturbances in the normal vaginal flora which predispose the mare to fungal endometritis. Thus, the authors' preference is to use antibiotics systemically whenever is possible. In this case, antibiotics that reach high levels in the endometrium and uterine lumen are selected. **Tables 2** and **3** list the common antibiotics used to treat mares with endometritis.

Correction of Anatomic Defects

Mares presenting anatomic defects in the reproductive tract should have these abnormalities surgically corrected before breeding. The most common anatomic defects observed are poor perineal conformation, poor opposition of vulvar lips or lacerations to the perineal body. Lacerations of the perineal body are often underdiagnosed and this is one of the common problems we encounter in referral cases of subfertile mares in our practice. This defect can be easily fixed with a simple surgical procedure as shown in **Fig. 5**. If mare is confirmed to have a cervical laceration, pending on the size and location, the mare may need to undergo surgery. It has been the authors' experience that if the vaginal portion of the cervical is lacerated most mares are able to carry and delivery normal pregnancies without the need to fix the cervix. On

Table 2
Drugs commonly used for intrauterine infusion in mares

Drug	Dosage	Comments
Amikacin sulfate	1–2 g	Buffer with equal volume of 7.5% NaHCO3 or large volume (150–200 mL)
Ampicillin	1–2 g	Gram-negative spectrum, use soluble product at high dilution, may be irritating when concentrated; susceptible gram-positive and gram-negative organisms, including E. coli
Ceftiofur sodium	1 g	Broad spectrum (S zooepidemicus), reserve for organisms resistant to other antimicrobials; susceptible gram-negative and gram-positive organisms
Gentamicin sulfate	1–2 g	Buffer with NaHCO3 or large volume (150–200 mL) saline solution; susceptible S zooepidemicus (some isolates), Enterobacter spp, E coli, Klebsiella spp, Proteus spp, Serratia spp, P aeruinosa, S aureus
Neomycin sulfate	2–4 g	Gram-negative spectrum, useful against E coli and some Klebsiella spp
Potassium penicillin	5 million units	Gram positive spectrum (S zooepidemicus)
Polymyxin B	1 million units	Good spectrum against Pseudomonas spp
Ticarcillin	3–6 g	Anti-pseudomonas; β-lactam drug; good spectrum against gram-positive organisms; infuse diluted in a minimum of 200 mL of saline solution
Ticarcillin	3–6 g	Clavulanic acid is a β-lactamase inhibitor, confers greater activity against Enterobacter spp, S aureus, Bacillus fragillis, S zooepidemicus; infuse with a minimum of 150–200 mL saline solution

Data from Canisso IF, Coutinho da Silva MA. Bacterial endometritis. Sprayberry KA, Robinson NE, editors. In: Robinson's current therapy in equine medicine. St Louis (MO): WB Saunders; 2015. p. 683–88.

Table 3
Commonly used systemic antimicrobials for endometritis in mares

Antimicrobial	Dosage	Route
Amikacin sulfate	10 mg/kg q24 h	IV or IM
Ampicillin	29 mg/kg q12 or 24 h	IV or IM
Ceftiofur sodium	2.5 mg/kg q12–24 h	IV or IM
Ceftiofur crystalline free acid	6.6 mg/kg q4 d	IM
Enrofloxacin	5 mg/kg q24 h	IV
	7.5 mg/kg q24 h	PO
Gentamicin sulfate	6.6 mg/kg q24 h	IV
Metronidazole	15–25 mg/kg	PO
Potassium penicillin	25,000 IU/kg q6 h	IV
Procaine penicillin	22,000 IU/kg q12 h	IM
Trimethoprim-sulfamethoxazole	30 mg/kg q12 h	PO

Data from Canisso IF, Coutinho da Silva MA. Bacterial endometritis. Sprayberry KA, Robinson NE, editors. In: Robinson's current therapy in equine medicine. St Louis (MO): WB Saunders; 2015. p. 683–88.

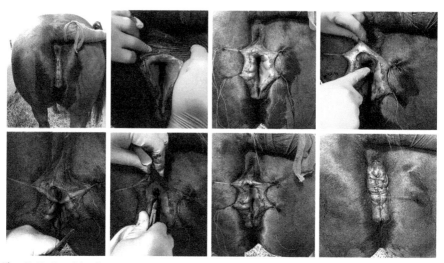

Fig. 5. Perineal body reconstruction in a Quarter Horse mare following a mild dystocia. After the mare is blocked with lidocaine, stay sutures are placed and then a flap of the dorsal aspect of the vestibule is removed, thereafter, the borders of the incision are sutured together to form a shelf and then the dorsal aspect closed with simple interrupted absorbable suture. The procedure is finished by placing Caslick's stitches.

the other hand, if the laceration is cranial in the cervix and extensive, surgical correction may not be possible.

Uterine Lavage

Uterine lavage is commonly used to manage endometritis in mares post-breeding. Obvious advantages include physical removal of microorganisms, sperm cells, debris, inflammatory products which may prolong the endometrial inflammation. Lactated Ringer's Solution (LRS) is the preferred and most commonly used solution to perform uterine flushing. Mucolytics and chelators can be used to improve uterine lavage (**Table 4**). In a typical post-breeding uterine lavage, 2 L are usually sufficient, but sometimes three to 5 L may be necessary. While performing uterine lavage, the practitioner needs to ensure that the entire uterus is fully distended to ensure that the whole surface is flushed, and the lavage is continued until the effluent is clear.

Maiden mares will typically tolerate 1 L of LRS at the time, and broodmares can easily tolerate 2 L of LRS in their uteri. It is worth noting that some mares may present signs of mild discomfort (shifting weight, moving hind legs up and body forward) when 2 L of LRS are used. However, the use of 2 L of LRS per flush assures that the entire uterus is dilated and flushed and facilitates fluid recovery.

Post-breeding uterine lavage is commonly performed with a Bivona-type catheter, and the balloon inflated to avoid reflux of fluid through the cervix. This procedure is first performed 6 to 24 hours post-breeding, and repeated daily, if necessary, until deemed no longer necessary. Mares presenting intra-uterine fluid accumulation pre-breeding may have uterine lavage performed immediately prior to breeding. The criteria for lavaging a mare's uterus pre- and post-breeding can be based on the mare's history of producing excessive amounts of fluid post-breeding, the detection of moderate to large amounts of intrauterine fluid accumulation (>2 cm depth) with certain defining features (ie, intrauterine fluid accumulation with high echogenicity), or simply clinician's preference.

Table 4
Other treatments used in mares with endometritis

Product	Mechanism of Action	Comments
Dimethyslsulfoxide (DMSO 10%–20%)	Postulated to reduce endometrial inflammation by scavenging free radical	May result in irritation if applied in high concentration
N-acetylcysteine (5%–10% solution)	Postulated to disrupt disulfide bonds between polymers, resulting in clearance	Anecdotally effective in improving pregnancy rates for barren mares with history of bacterial endometritis
Buffered chelators (Tris EDTA and Tricide)	Postulated to chelate divalent cations in the fungal cell membrane, resulting in altered fungal structural integrity	Potentiates the effects of antifungals and decreases resistance to antifungals

Data from Canisso IF, Coutinho da Silva MA. Bacterial endometritis. Sprayberry KA, Robinson NE, editors. In: Robinson's current therapy in equine medicine. St Louis (MO): WB Saunders; 2015. p. 683–88.

We prefer to perform uterine lavage by 6 hours post breeding. It is our clinical experience that flushing the uterine lumen at this time helps to avoid excessive inflammatory response in susceptible mares. Our anecdotal experiences are supported by controlled design studies where the authors found that 6 hours post-breeding appears to be a critical time point for uterine inflammation between susceptible and resistant mares.[17,23] Additionally, sperm transport appears to be completed by 4 hours post-breeding,[37] and fertility should not be affected by uterine lavage performed at or after 4 hours post-breeding.[38] As a basic rule, when performing uterine lavage, additional flushing should be added if the last fluid recovered still appears cloudy and/or contain mucus strings (**Fig. 6**).

Ecbolic

Oxytocin and cloprostenol (an analog of prostaglandin F 2 α (PGF2α)) have been commonly used as ecbolic agents. These drugs stimulate uterine contractility and eliminate intrauterine fluid accumulation through an open cervix and/or through lymphatic drainage. Oxytocin is associated with strong uterine contractions for a short period of time (<45 min); whereas cloprostenol (125–250 mcg/IM) induces a weak but prolonged uterine contraction (up to 2 h).[10,39] In our clinical experience prolonged uterine contraction appears to be very beneficial for mares with a very pendulous uterus.

We recommend to begin oxytocin therapy by 6 hours post breeding or pre-breeding if the mare has intrauterine fluid accumulation. Oxytocin (20 units/IM) is administered at intervals of 2 to 8 hours. In our practice, susceptible mares may receive oxytocin every 2 hours. We only use needles with very small calibers, typically a 25 gauge needle, to prevent a mare from becoming needle-shy or aggressive toward the person administering the drugs. Smaller doses of oxytocin (10–20 units) are more effective in inducing uterine contractions than larger doses (40 units), as larger doses induce tetanic uterine contractions rather than cyclic uterine contractions, thus preventing uterine evacuation.[10]

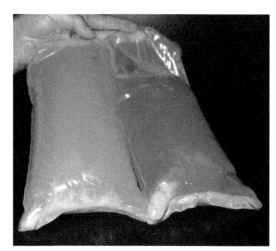

Fig. 6. Severe inflammatory response in a mare highly susceptible to endometritis. This uterine lavage was performed approximately 6 to 8 h post-insemination. The second bag of fluid (on right) contains less debris; however, flush was continued until effluent was clear.

Cloprostenol should be used with caution as it may be associated with hemorrhagic anovulatory follicles and is therefore not recommended in older mares with history of HAF.[40] Additionally, cloprostenol should not be given to mares post-ovulation because it will interfere with CL formation and progesterone secretion.[39]

Carbetocin, a long-acting oxytocin analog, has been introduced as a potentially more effective alternative to oxytocin[41] or cloprostenol in the breeding management of mares. However, its use in clinical practice has been rather limited and more data is needed before specific recommendations regarding its use can be provided.

Prostaglandin E & Misoprostol

Old maiden mares, nervous young maiden mares, and embryo donor mares (used for embryo donation without carrying foals to term), are very likely to present excessive post-breeding fluid accumulation due to inadequate cervical dilation during estrus. The authors recommend managing such mares proactively by performing uterine lavage 6 hours post breeding. Moreover, prostaglandin E preparations or misoprostol can be applied on the cervix after uterine lavage to maintain the cervix open. Such mares may also have the cervix gently dilated manually during the lavage. Some clinicians advocate drawing of the uterine catheter from the uterus with the balloon inflated to help stretch the cervix.

Prostaglandin E may be purchased as a cream/liquid preparation from compounding pharmacies or human pharmacy and can be applied directly to the cervix (2–2.5 mg/mare). In addition to not being readily available as a commercial product, another major disadvantage of this drug is the elevated cost, making it not feasible to use on all mares. This is in contrast to misoprostol (a synthetic prostaglandin E1 analogue), which is inexpensive and widely available as 100 mcg tablets that can be crushed, mixed with sterile lube, and directly applied to the cervix. The recommended dose for this treatment is 1 to 2 mg/mare. However, it is worth to note that a recent controlled study did not find measureable differences in mares receiving 1 mg intracervically.[42] In our practice, we associate the use of misoprostol with manual dilation of the cervix and which appears to enhance its response. Another controversial treatment that has been described to relax the cervix in susceptible mare is buscopan. Some clinicians advocate using buscopan (N-butylscopolammonium bromide 20 mg/mL) 20 to 40 mg locally in the cervical lumen to aid in stretching the cervix. The authors' have used buscopan with variable results, but currently no controlled data is available to justify its use.

Uteropexy

In Thoroughbreds, assisted reproductive techniques are not allowed, which represents a challenge to those mares that may have difficulties conceiving due to the presence of a pendulous uterus. With that in mind, Brink and collaborators[43] described a surgical technique using laparoscopy to imbricate the mesometrium in 5 barren mares. Three out of five mares became pregnant within the same year without any major intervention. Standard abdominal laparoscopic technique is performed under sedation with the mare standing in stocks. The dorsal aspect of the mesometrium and myometrium and perimetrium are then sutured together by a simple continuous suture placed 1.5 cm apart (10–14 bites per side). Though the technique has potential to improve reproduction in the Thoroughbred industry, it does not seem to be widely utilized for unknown reasons. We speculate that this underutilization may be due to financial constraints of the owners or that most clinicians are unfamiliar with the technique. Regardless, this technique should be considered as a viable option when indicated.

Breeding Management

Most clinicians' agree that susceptible mares should be bred with highly fertile semen whenever possible, and some advocate to breed the mare several days from ovulation to allow time for the uterine inflammation to subside before the embryo enters the uterus. Susceptible mares can have semen deposited in the uterine body as deep horn insemination, with frozen or fresh cooled semen, using either a flexible AI pipette or hysteroscopy; however, this was associated with lower pregnancy rates in susceptible mares, in contrast to enhanced pregnancy rates in resistant mares.[44] Moreover, mares should be inseminated only once per cycle, in order to decrease the inflammatory stimulus to the endometrium. Thus, the use of ovulation inducing agents is indicated, such as deslorelin acetate (1.8 mg) or human chorionic gonadotropin (1500–2500 Units).

Immune Modulators

Glucocorticoids are the most widely used immunomodulatory drugs to manage mares susceptible to endometritis. Recently, non-traditional immunomodulatory agents such as platelet-rich plasma, mycobacterium cell wall extract, Propionibacterium acnes, and Ceragyn have also been used to manage mares with variable success, and these therapies are being covered in Charles F. Scoggin's article, "Endometritis: Non-Traditional Therapies," in this issue.

Administration of prednisone acetate starting 2 days before breeding was effective in improving pregnancy rates in mares bred with frozen semen.[45] Intravenous administration of 50 mg dexamethasone ($\sim$0.1 mg/kg) within 1 hour of breeding in combination with common treatment (ecbolics, uterine lavage) reduced persistent post-breeding endometritis as assessed by decreasing post-mating efflux turbidity and endometrial edema with no change in the number of PMN cells recovered by small volume lavage.[46] Interesting to note that dexamethasone only improved pregnancy rates in mares presenting with more than three risk factors (see **Table 1**).[46] This study demonstrated the importance of case selection when deciding to give dexamethasone to mares at breeding time. In our practice, we typically administer 20 to 40 mg

(IV) to mares with history of excessive intrauterine fluid accumulation around breeding and may repeat the dose at 24 hours after breeding if the mare is presenting excessive intrauterine fluid accumulation. However, other authors failed to observe improvement in pregnancy rates in ~700 cycles of ~350 treated with 10 to 20 mg of dexamethasone.[47]

Uterine inflammation post-breeding is a physiologic reaction of the endometrium to sperm that subsides in 24 to 48 h. Persistence of this inflammatory reaction beyond 48 h is caused by many different factors alone or in association. Thus, the clinical approach to manage cases of persistent post-breeding endometritis should be based on the reproductive characteristics of the individual mare and adapted to circumvent or improve these faults, in order to maximize pregnancy and foaling rates.

REFERENCES

1. Traub-Dargatz JL, Salman MD, Voss JL. Medical problems of adult horses, as ranked by equine practitioners. J Am Vet Med Assoc 1991;198(10):1745–7.
2. Riddle WT, LeBlanc MM, Stromberg AJ. Relationships between uterine culture, cytology and pregnancy rates in a Thoroughbred practice. Theriogenology 2007;8(68):395–402.
3. Watson DE. Post breeding endometritis in the mare. Anim Reprod Sci 2000; 60-61:221–32.
4. Hurtgen JP. Pathogenesis and treatment of endometritis in the mare: a review. Theriogenology 2006;66:560–6.
5. Troedsson MHT. Breeding-induced endometritis in mares. Vet Clin North Am Equine Pract 2006;22:705–12.
6. Hughes JP, Loy RG. Investigations on the effect on intrauterine inoculation of Streptococcus zooepidemicus in the mare. Proc Am Assoc Equine Pract 1969; 15:289–92.
7. Zent WW, Troedsson MHT, Xue JL. Postbreeding uterine fluid accumulation in a normal population of Thoroughbred mares: a field study. Proc Am Assoc Equine Pract 1998;44:64–5.
8. Troedsson MH, Loset K, Alghamdi AM, et al. Interaction between equine semen and the endometrium: the inflammatory response to semen. Anim Reprod Sci 2001;68:273–9.
9. Troedsson MHT, Steiger BN, Ibrahim NM, et al. Mechanism of sperm induced endometritis in the mare. Biol Reprod Mono 1995;52(supp I):307 [abstract].
10. Troedsson MHT, Liu IKM, Ing M, et al. Smooth muscle electrical activity in the oviduct and the effect of oxytocin, PG2α, PGE2 on the myometrium and oviduct of the cycling mare. Biol Reprod Mono 1995;1:439–52.
11. Katila T. Onset and duration of uterine inflammatory response of mares after insemination with fresh semen. Biol Reprod Mono 1995;1:515–7.
12. Troedsson MH, Desvousges A, Alghamdi AS, et al. Components in seminal plasma regulating sperm transport and elimination. Anim Reprod Sci 2005;89: 171–86.
13. Alghamdi AS, Foster DN. Seminal DNase frees spermatozoa entangled in neutrophil extracellular traps. Biol Reprod 2005;73:1174–81.
14. Rebordão M, Carneiro C, Alexandre-Pires G, et al. Neutrophil extracellular traps formation by bacteria causing endometritis in the mare. J Reprod Immunol 2014; 106:41–9.

15. Galvao A, Rebordao MR, Szostekc AZ, et al. Cytokines and neutrophil extracellular traps in the equine endometrium: friends or foes? Pferdeheilkunde 2012; 28:4–7.
16. Katila T, Sankari S, Makela O. Transport of spermatozoa in the reproductive tracts of mares. J Reprod Fertil Suppl 2000;56:571–8.
17. Troedsson MH, Woodward EM. Our current understanding of the pathophysiology of equine endometritis with an emphasis on breeding-induced endometritis. Reprod Biol 2016;16:8–12.
18. LeBlanc M, Neuwirth L, Mauragis D, et al. Oxytocin enhances clearance of radiocolloid from the uterine lumen of reproductively normal mares and mares susceptible to endometritis. Equine Vet J 1994;26:279–82.
19. LeBlanc MM, Neuwirth L, Jones L, et al. Differences in uterine position of the reproductively normal mares and those with delayed uterine clearance detected by scintigraphy. Theriogenology 1998;50:49–50.
20. Alghamdi AS, Foster DN, Carlson CS, et al. Nitric oxide levels and nitric oxide synthase expression in uterine samples from mares susceptible and resistant to persistent breeding-induced endometritis. Am J Reprod Immunol 2005;53: 230–7.
21. Woodward EM, Christoffersen M, Campos J, et al. Endometrial inflammatory markers of the early immune response in mares susceptible or resistant to persistent breeding-induced endometritis. Reproduction 2013;145:289–96.
22. Forshey BS, Messerschmidt CA, Pinto CRF, et al. Effects of lactoferrin on postbreeding uterine inflammation in the mare. Clin Theriogenol 2011;3:363.
23. Woodward EM, Troedsson MH. Equine breeding-induced endometritis: a review. J Equine Vet Sci 2013;33(9):673–82.
24. Rasmussen CD, Morten PR, Bojesen AM, et al. Equine infectious endometritis-clinical and subclinical cases. J Equine Vet Sci 2015;35:95–104.
25. Cocchia N, Paciello O, Auletta L, et al. Comparison of the cytobrush, cottonswab, and low-volume uterine flush techniques to evaluate endometrial cytology for diagnosing endometritis in chronically infertile mares. Theriogenology 2012;77: 89–98.
26. Overbeck W, Witte TS, Heuwieser W. Comparison of three diagnostic methods to identify subclinical endometritis in mares. Theriogenology 2011;75:1311–8.
27. Davies Morel MC, Lawlor O, Nash DM. Equine endometrial cytology and bacteriology: effectiveness for predicting live foaling rates. Vet J 2013;198:206–11.
28. LeBlanc MM, Magsig J, Stromberg AJ. Use of a low-volume uterine flush for diagnosing endometritis in chronically infertile mares. Theriogenology 2007;68: 403–12.
29. Nielsen JM. Endometritis in the mare: a diagnostic study comparing cultures from swab and biopsy. Theriogenology 2005;64:510–8.
30. Christoffersen M, Brandis L, Samuelsson J, et al. Diagnostic double-guarded low-volume uterine lavage in mares. Theriogenology 2015;83:222–7.
31. Kenney RM, Doig PA. Equine endometrial biopsy. Current therapy in theriogenology. Philadelphia: WB Saunders; 1986. p. 723–9.
32. Waelchi RO. Endometrial biopsy in mares under nonuniform breeding management conditions: prognostic value and relationship with age. Can Vet J 1990; 31:379–84.
33. Nielsen JM, Nielsen FH, Petersen MR. Diagnosis of equine endometritis – microbiology, cytology, and histology of endometrial biopsies and the correlation to fertility. Pferdeheilkunde 2012;28:8–13.

34. Barbacini S, Necchi D, Zavaglia G, et al. Retrospective study on the incidence of post insemination uterine fluid in mares inseminated with frozen/thawed semen. J Equine Vet Sci 2003;23(11):493–6.

35. Brinsko SP, Rigby SL, Varner DD, et al. A practical method for recognizing mares susceptible to post-breeding endometritis. Proc Am Assoc Equine Pract 2003;49: 363–5.

36. Canisso IF, Coutinho da Silva MA. Bacterial endometritis. In: Sprayberry KA, Robinson NE, editors. Robinson's current therapy in equine medicine. St Louis (MO): WB Saunders; 2015. p. 683–8.

37. Scott MA. A glimpse at sperm function in vivo: sperm transport and epithelial interaction in the female reproductive tract. Anim Reprod Sci 2000;60-61:337–48.

38. Brinsko SP, Varner DD, Blanchard TL. The effect of uterine lavage performed four hours post insemination on pregnancy rate in mares. Theriogenology 1991;35: 1111–9.

39. Troedsson MH, Ababneh MM, Ohlgren AF, et al. Effect of periovulatory prostaglandin Falpah on pregnancy rates and luteal function in the mare. Theriogenology 2001;55:1891–9.

40. Cuervo-Arango J, Newcombe JR. Risk factors for the development of haemorrhagic anovulatory follicles in the mare. Reprod Domest Anim 2010;45:473–80.

41. Stecker D, Naidoo V, Gerber D, et al. Ex vivo influence of carbetocin on equine myometrial muscles and comparison with oxytocin. Theriogenology 2012;78: 502–9.

42. McNaughten J, Pozor M, Macpherson M, et al. Effects of topical application of misoprostol on cervical relaxation in mares. Reprod Domest Anim 2014;49: 1057–62.

43. Brink P, Schumacher J, Schumacher J. Elevating the uterus (uteropexy) of five mares by laparoscopically imbricating the mesometrium. Equine Vet J 2010;42: 675–9.

44. Sieme H, Bonk A, Hamann H, et al. Effects of different artificial insemination techniques and sperm doses on fertility of normal mares and mares with abnormal reproductive history. Theriogenology 2004;62:915–28.

45. Dell'Aqua JA Jr, Papa FO, Lopes MD, et al. Modulation of acute uterine inflammatory response after artificial insemination with equine frozen semen. Anim Reprod Sci 2006;94:270–3.

46. Bucca S, Carli A, Buckley T, et al. The use of dexamethasone administered to mares at breeding time in the modulation of persistent mating induced endometritis. Theriogenology 2008;70:1093–100.

47. Vandale H, Daels P, Piepers S, et al. Effect of post-insemination dexamethasone treatment on pregnancy rates in mares. Anim Reprod Sci 2010;121S:S110–2.

Endometritis

Diagnostic Tools for Infectious Endometritis

Ryan A. Ferris, DVM, MS

KEYWORDS

- Bacterial • Fungal • Endometritis • Diagnostics • Interpretation

KEY POINTS

- Detection of infectious endometritis is challenging.
- No single diagnostic test is capable of detecting all cases of infectious endometritis.
- A guarded swab and cytology brush can be used as initial screening diagnostics to be analyzed by microbial culture and cytologic evaluation diagnosis of infectious endometritis.
- If results from the initial screening testing are negative for mares with clinical signs suggestive of infectious endometritis, additional samples collected by small-volume lavage or uterine biopsy should be submitted for microbial culture and cytologic evaluation.

Infectious endometritis is among the leading causes of subfertility in the mare.[1,2] However, the best way to reliably diagnose these cases of infectious endometritis can be confusing to the veterinary practitioner. The goal of this article is to describe how to perform various sample collection techniques, what analysis can be performed on these samples, and how to interpret the results of these analysis. Additionally, future technologies will be presented that are not currently used in equine reproduction practice.

INTRODUCTION

Infectious endometritis is reported as among the top problems equine practitioners face in clinical practice.[1] Risk factors for developing infectious endometritis include

- Failure to become pregnant or donate an embryo after 3 breeding cycles to a fertile stallion
- Less than two-thirds of the vulva below the brim of the pelvis
- Poor or decreased muscular tone to the vulva

The author has nothing to disclose.
Equine Reproduction Laboratory, Department of Clinical Sciences, Colorado State University, 3101 Rampart Road, Fort Collins, CO 80521, USA
E-mail address: rferris@colostate.edu

Vet Clin Equine 32 (2016) 481–498
http://dx.doi.org/10.1016/j.cveq.2016.08.001
0749-0739/16/Published by Elsevier Inc.

- Poor conformation to the perineum
- Cervical abnormalities (trauma, adhesions, fibrosis)
- Abnormalities of the vulva (trauma)
- Decreased uterine contractility
- Exposure to pathogens during breeding
- Chronic intrauterine antibiotic administration
- Pendulous uterus
- Windsucking–aspiration of air into the reproductive tract
- Equine pituitary pars intermedia dysfunction
- Poor body condition (body condition score <4 out of 9)

Normally, the mare's uterus can rapidly clear infections if exposed to bacteria or fungal organisms. However, any breakdown in the defense mechanisms of the reproductive tract will predispose a mare to a uterine infection such as

- Conformation—abnormalities of the perineum, vestibulo–vaginal seal, or cervix may allow increased numbers of pathogens to reach the uterus
- Uterine clearance—decreased ability of the mare's uterus to contract, reducing clearance of fluid and contaminants from the uterus
- Innate immune system—breakdown in the response toward pathogens in the uterus
- Exposure during breeding to a venereal pathogen

During routine evaluations of the mare, the mare common findings that strongly suggest infectious endometritis and warrant additional diagnostics include

- Large volume or echogenic fluid in the uterine lumen during estrus[3]
- Excessive uterine edema
- Any fluid present in the uterine lumen in diestrus
- Hyperemic cervix with or without a discharge from the cervical os

Once a case of infectious endometritis is suspected, the next decision facing the equine clinician is what samples to collect and what analysis to perform on the collected samples. Commonly, a review of uterine culture and cytology is performed, evaluating the uterus for the presence of infectious organisms (**Box 1**), common organisms cultured from the equine reproductive tract, or white blood cells (WBCs) in the uterine lumen. Additional advanced or confirmatory tests can be performed such as a small-volume lavage or uterine biopsy.

The equine clinician relies on the diagnostic techniques to determine if a particular mare is affected by infectious endometritis. These diagnostics are routinely performed in practice to both diagnose and rule out infectious endometritis as a cause of the observed subfertility.

Collection of Samples from the Equine Uterus

Preparation of the mare

The tail of the mare should be wrapped and held out of the way to minimize contamination potential of the mare's reproductive tract and the collection sample. The perineal area should be washed with a nonresidual soap and rinsed with clean water a minimum of 3 times or sufficiently to remove all external debris. The region should be dried with disposable paper towels. A small moist piece of paper towel should be used to gently wipe the inside of the vestibule to remove fecal material and debris that could otherwise be inadvertently transferred into the uterus during sample collection. This should be performed from the dorsal to ventral commissure to prevent contamination from the clitoral fossa.

Box 1
Common bacteria and fungal organisms cultured from the equine uterus

- Etiologic agents detected in the equine uterus
- Bacteria known to be pathogenic
  - *Streptococcus* species
    - β-hemolytic
    - Equi subspecies zooepidemicus
  - *Escherichia coli*
  - *Pseudomonas* species
    - Aeruginosa
    - Fluorescens
  - *Klebsiella* species
    - Pneumoniae
- Bacteria with questionable pathogenicity
  - Methicillin-resistant *Staphlococcus aureus*
  - *Streptococcus* species
    - α-hemolytic
    - Nonhemolytic
    - Faecalis
    - Equisimilis
  - *Bordetella bronchiseptica*
  - *Proteus* species
    - Mirabilis
    - Vulgaris
  - *Staphylococcus* species
    - Aureus
    - Albus
    - Intermedius
  - *Serratia* species
  - *Corynebacterium* species
  - *Citrobacter* species
  - *Enterobacter* species
  - *Bacillus* species
  - *Actinetobacter* species
  - *Micrococcus* species
  - *Pasturella* species
  - Anaerobic
  - *Bacteroides fragilis*
  - *Fusobacterium* species
  - *Clostridium* species
    - Perfringens
    - Difficile
  - *Mycoplasma* subspecies
  - *Chlamydia* subspecies
- Fungal organisms
  - *Candida* species
    - Albicans
    - Other
  - *Aspergillus* species
  - *Actinomyces* species
    - Fumigatus
  - *Cryptococcus* species
  - *Fusarium* species
  - *Mucor* species

Guarded swab

Commonly, a guarded swab is used for collection of a sample for submission for bacterial or fungal growth and to obtain a sample of the cells on the surface of the endometrial surface or in the uterine lumen. For microbiology culture, the swab is advanced by the clinician through the mare's cervix into the uterine lumen and left in contact with the endometrial surface for 20 to 30 seconds. The swab is retracted back into the guard and removed from the reproductive tract of the mare. The swab can be placed into transport media (Amies liquid media or similar) until the swab is submitted to the laboratory for analysis. Alternatively, the swab can be immediately plated onto agar plates (discussed in detail) for bacterial or fungal growth. For a cytology sample, the swab is gently rolled onto a glass slide, and the glass slide is allowed to air dry for future evaluation.

A swab may not be the best diagnostic sample due to increased cellular damage and decreased diagnostic capability.[4-6] A study showed that the sensitivity of a swab for diagnosing inflammation in the uterus was dramatically lower (0.00) compared with cytology brush (0.17).[5]

Guarded cytology brush

The guarded cytology brush (**Fig. 1**A) provides a sample with better cellularity and minimal artifacts from the collection process compared with a sample collected from a swab.[4-7] The sample collection process is identical to the guarded swab. The cytology brush has been shown to have a higher sensitivity compared with a swab for diagnosing inflammation in the uterine lumen.[4-7] The guarded swab, while advantageous for collection of a cytology sample, has reduced sensitivity compared with a swab sample for the detection of microbial organisms (0.25 and 0.33, respectively).[5]

Single swab

A single guarded swab is preferred by some practitioners to collect a sample for culture using the swab; the cap of the swab is used to obtain a sample for cytology (**Fig. 1**B). It should be noted that there is potential for contamination of the cytology sample with cells and debris from the cervix and vagina during withdrawal of the

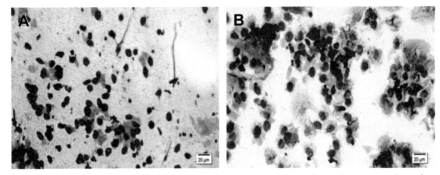

Fig. 1. Comparison of a guarded brush cytology versus a low volume lavage cytology from the same mare (40× objective). The brush cytology sample (*A*) contains a large number of individual and rafts of uterine epithelial cells. The low volume lavage sample (*B*) contains a concentrated number of cells per same high-power field. Artifacts from the centrifugation and processing steps, most notably disruption of the cytoplasm of UECs, can be noted on the LVL sample. (*From* Ferris RA, Bohn A, McCue PM. Equine endometrial cytology: collection techniques and interpretation. Equine Vet Educ 2015;27(6):316–22.)

instrument. Contamination can be reduced by guarding the cap in the vaginal vault with one's hand to limit vaginal contamination.

Collection of samples via speculum

Another common method to collect an endometrial cytology sample is to pass a swab or brush through a sterile disposable vaginal speculum and subsequently through the cervix for uterine sample collection.[8,9] This is especially advantageous in mares with a Caslick episioplasty that inhibits passage of the clinician's hand into the vaginal vault of the mare. It is recommended that this be done while the mare is in estrus to facilitate passage of the swab and diagnostic capabilities.[10]

The initial database should consist of both a uterine culture and cytology sample. Individually, a uterine culture or cytology has a low sensitivity for the diagnosis of infectious endometritis.[5,11] However, when a positive culture or cytology sample is used to determine a positive case of infectious endometritis, the sensitivity is improved to 0.42.[5] Depending on the causative infectious organism, the cytology results may change (eg, *Streptococcus zooepidemicus* is typically associated with a positive cytology sample as compared to *Escherichia coli*, which is typically associated with a cytology sample negative for inflammatory cells).[12] Additionally, a positive culture or cytology should be considered diagnostic of infectious endometritis, as these results are associated with reduced pregnancy rates.[11–13] Because of these findings, it is suggested that the minimal database for evaluation of infectious endometritis be both a guarded swab for microbial culture and a guarded cytology brush for cytologic evaluation.

A limiting factor with all swab or brush collection protocols is the fact that the sample is obtained from a small percentage of the endometrial surface or uterine lumen, and the sample may not be representative of the entire uterus. A clinical tip to improve the diagnostic capability of the swab or brush is that if uterine fluid is detected on ultrasound examination prior to collection of the sample, the swab and brush should be extremely wet with this fluid. If the swab and brush are relatively dry, the sample may not have been in the fluid, and a second sample should be collected.

Advanced or Confirmatory Collection Methods

The initial database is often used as a simple screening method for infectious endometritis. However, it is recognized that there will be false-negative samples with the guarded swab/brush technique. In mares strongly suspected of infectious endometritis that have no growth from a guarded swab and no evidence of inflammatory cells on cytology, additional diagnostic tests are warranted.

Small volume lavage

A low volume lavage may be performed in problem mares to provide a more complete sampling of the entire uterine lumen.[14,15] A volume of 150 mLs of sterile saline or lactated Ringer solution (LRS) is infused into the uterus by gravity flow. The fluid is gently massaged throughout the uterine lumen by palpation per rectum. The infused fluid is recovered by gravity flow after lowering the original fluid bag to ground level. Recovery is facilitated by transrectal massage of the uterus and intravenous administration of 20 units of oxytocin. Uterine effluent fluid is transferred into 1 or 2 sterile 50 mL conical tubes and centrifuged at $600 \times g$ for 10 minutes. The supernatant is aspirated or decanted, and the pellet can be submitted for microbiology culture, picked up with a cotton-tipped swab, and gently rolled onto a glass slide for cytologic evaluation (see **Fig. 1**B) or other advanced diagnostic tests. Alternatively, the pellet can be resuspended in a small amount of supernatant and a portion of this spread between 2 slides using a slide-on-slide technique.[16] There is often an increase in cellular artifacts (eg, damaged or disrupted cells) associated with the centrifugation process versus samples collected by uterine swab or brush. The fluid and processing techniques associated with a low volume lavage sample had no effect on the quality or diagnostic capabilities of the resulting cytology smear.[4]

The use of the small volume lavage for the diagnosis of infectious endometritis results in an improved sensitivity for culture of 0.71 and cytology of 0.80. The improved sensitivity with this technique results in fewer false-negative samples as compared to a guarded swab or brush cytology sample. However, increased time and personnel required to perform a small volume lavage have prevented this diagnostic technique from replacing a traditional guarded culture and cytology as the initial diagnostic technique to screen for infectious endometritis.

Endometrial biopsy

An equine endometrial biopsy instrument is passed manually, with the jaws in the closed position, through the vestibule, vagina, and cervix into the uterine lumen. Once the basket of the instrument is in the uterine lumen, the hand is removed from the reproductive tract and passed per rectum over the site where the jaws are located. The punch is rotated so the jaws are positioned horizontally and the handle released, opening the jaws. The endometrium is pressed firmly into the jaws, closed, and the tissue is excised and removed. The tissue can be placed into a fixative for histologic evaluation, submitted for microbial culture; impression smears may also be made to interpret a cytology sample.

To fix the tissue, the sample should be immediately immersed in Bouin solution; after 12 to 24 hours of fixation, the tissue is removed and placed in 70% ethanol to prevent further hardening of the tissue. The sample should be submitted for histologic processing and evaluation by personnel experienced with interpreting equine endometrial samples.

Histologic evaluation of the endometrium for the presence of WBCs in the stratum compactum has been used as the gold standard for diagnosing infectious endometritis.[13,17–20]

Culture of an endometrial biopsy has resulted in improved sensitivity (0.82) compared with a guarded swab (0.34).[13] In cases in which the endometrial cytology was positive, there were less negative microbial culture from a uterine biopsy (3%) compared with a guarded swab (26%).[13] These data suggest that bacteria may be present deep within the glands of the endometrium and not as commonly on the surface of the endometrium.

Evaluation of Samples

Microbiology

For many equine reproduction practitioners, microbiology can be frustrating. By the time a culture is taken, sent to a laboratory, and the results reported, the mare has already ovulated, and the window of time for directed intervention has passed for that cycle. Likewise, the prospect of performing in-house microbiology can seem overwhelming, time-consuming, and tedious. The reality is that in-house microbiology can be practical, simple, and inexpensive.

Samples should be applied to agar that is capable of supporting growth of common equine uterine pathogens. Common agar that has been utilized for cultivating equine uterine bacterial pathogens are trypticase soy agar (TSA) with 5% sheep blood, MacConkey agar, and chromogenic agar.[21,22] Sabouraud agar is routinely used for the cultivation of fungal organisms; often this agar contains chloramphenicol to prevent bacterial overgrowth. Approximately 1% to 5% of uterine swabs submitted to a diagnostic laboratory are positive for fungal growth.[23]

The swab pellet from a small volume lavage or uterine biopsy should be applied directly to the agar surface and streaked back and forth over approximately 30% to 50% of the agar surface (primary streak), with a flamed inoculation loop or sterile swab streak through the primary streak once. One should continue to streak the second third of the plate (secondary streak). Next, streak through the secondary streak once and continue to streak the final third of the plate (tertiary streak). The whole idea is to dilute or spread out the colonies so that individual colonies will be available to work with and identify. This allows for the amount of growth to be characterized and the resulting severity of the infection to be predicted (**Table 1**).

Initial results are available after 12 to 24 hours of cultivation, but plates should be monitored for 72 hours for the presence of slow-growing bacterial organisms or fungal pathogens. In the authors' clinical setting, this allows for the results of the microbiology culture to be known by 7 AM when mares start to be examined, allowing for these results to be considered when trying to optimize breeding management.

Bacterial isolates can be easily identified by their growth characteristics on common agar (**Figs. 2–5, Table 2**). Recent work in the authors' laboratory showed that uterine isolates of *Streptococcus zooepidemicus, E coli, Pseudomonas Aeruginosa,* and *Klebsiella pneumoniae* cultivated on TSA with 5% sheep blood, MacConkey agar, and a gram-positive/negative selective chromogenic agar were easily identified by untrained personnel based on comparison with common bacteria isolated from the equine uterus. Identification based on growth characteristics was 96% accurate as compared with 2 commercial identification systems (38% and 86%).

Antibiotic sensitivity (Kirby-Bauer method) can be done easily by selecting single colonies and streaking the bacteria onto Mueller Hinton agar and applying antibiotic discs directly to the agar surface. After 18 to 24 hours of cultivation, the zone of bacterial inhibition can be measured and susceptibility or resistance determined for that particular antibiotic (**Fig. 6**). This method allows the practitioner to screen for the common antibiotics that they use in clinical practice.

Cytology

Endometrial cytology is a rapid and inexpensive technique to detect the presence of endometritis. A diagnosis can often be made based on cytology results alone and suitable therapy initiated several days prior to obtaining results of microbial culture.

The glass slides with the sample applied from the previously mentioned cytology brush, small volume lavage pellet, or uterine biopsy are allowed to air dry and are stained with a modified Wright stain. If a prolonged period of time (>12 hours) is anticipated between collection and staining, a methanol or spray fixative can be used to

Table 1	
Determination of bacterial growth characteristic relative to the number of colonies of each organism present at 24 and 48 hours	
Growth	**Number of Colonies**
No growth	0
Very light	≤2, primary streak
Light	3–5, primary streak
Moderate	>5, into secondary streak
Heavy	>5, into tertiary streak

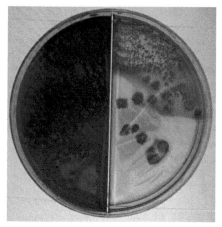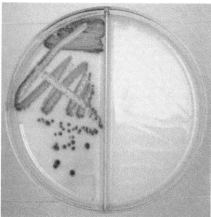

Fig. 2. Growth of *Escherichia coli* on agar plates; left image is a split plate of TSA with 5% sheep blood on the left and MacConkey agar on the right. The right image a selective chromogenic agar with a gram-negative selection on the left and a gram-positive selection on the right.

maintain cellular architecture. Additional stains that may be considered are a Gram stain or a fungus-specific stain such as Grocott Methenamine silver (GMS) stain.

Evaluation of uterine cytology slides should be thorough and systematic. An initial evaluation is performed at low magnification to determine if there is adequate cellularity to provide accurate interpretation. If the slide is determined to be of inadequate cellularity (ie, a low number of uterine epithelial cells or UECs) to be of diagnostic quality, a new sample should be collected.

If the sample is determined to be of diagnostic quality, the slide is then evaluated at 400× (10× eyepiece × 40× objective) magnification with multiple high power fields

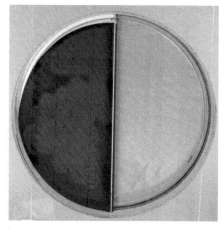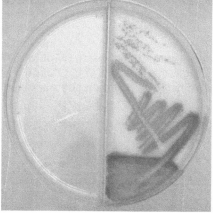

Fig. 3. Growth of *Streptococcus equi* subspecies *zooepidemicus* on agar plates; left image is a split plate of TSA with 5% sheep blood on the left and MacConkey agar on the right. The right image a selective chromogenic agar with a gram-negative selection on the left and a gram-positive selection on the right.

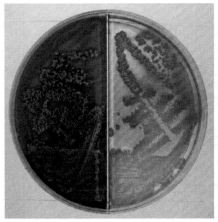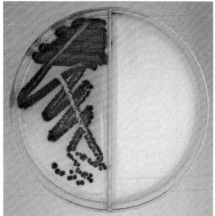

Fig. 4. Growth of *Klebsiella pneumoniae* on agar plates; left image is a split plate of TSA with 5% sheep blood on the left and MacConkey agar on the right. The right image a selective chromogenic agar with a gram-negative selection on the left and a gram-positive selection on the right.

examined for UECs (individual cells and rafts of cells), WBCs, debris, red blood cells, bacteria, yeast, fungal organisms, and spermatozoa. Evaluation of a field of view at 400× magnification is often referred to as a high power field (hpf). Evaluation at 1000× (10× eyepiece × 100× oil-immersion objective) magnification may be required to confirm the presence of bacterial and fungal pathogens detected at 400×. A check sheet can be utilized to rapidly and accurately record the observations.

Uterine epithelial cells Uterine epithelial cells can range from cuboidal in anestrus to tall columnar during the estrous cycle.[24] Most UECs are not ciliated, but ciliated cells are often observed in cytology preparations (**Fig. 7**). A range of UECs may be noted,

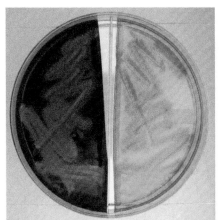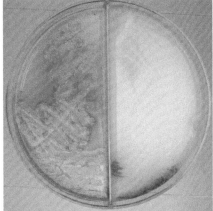

Fig. 5. Growth of *Pseudomonas aeruginosa* on agar plates; left image is a split plate of TSA with 5% sheep blood on the left and MacConkey agar on the right. The right image a selective chromogenic agar with a gram-negative selection on the left and a gram-positive selection on the right.

Table 2
Bacterial growth characteristics for deification of common equine uterine pathogens. Characteristics of chromogenic agar may only specific to Spectrum Agar, VetLabs

Organism	Gram Stain	Morph	TSA-5% Sheep Blood	MacConkey	Culture Characteristics Gram + Chromagar	Gram − Chromagar	Comments
Streptococcus zooepidemicus	Pos	Cocci, chains	Small, white, round colonies with beta hemolysis (0.5–1 mm)	No growth	Small, light blue colonies	No growth	Training is required to differentiate alpha and beta hemolysis
Escherichia coli	Neg	Rods	Cream to gray colored colonies ± alpha hemolysis (2–3 mm)	Medium sized, gray to pink colonies	No growth	Medium, pink to red colonies	
Klebsiella pneumoniae	Neg	Rods	Large gray mucoid colonies (2–4 mm)	Large, pink mucoid colonies	No Growth	Large, dark blue colonies with slight pink halo	Pink halo may take 24–36 h to develop and is faint
Pseudomonas aeruginosa	Neg	Rod	Flat metallic blue colonies (3–4 mm)	Large, pale greenish colonies	No growth	Transparent white to green colonies	"Grape-like" odor on blood agar, fluorescence with UV light
Staphylococcus aureus	Pos	Cocci, clusters	Medium, cream to gold colonies, +/− beta hemolysis (2–3 mm)	No growth or limited growth of pink colonies	White to yellow colonies	No growth	
Candida albicans			Soft, creamy raised, glistening colonies				Beer-like odor, suspect yeast if antibiotic sensitivity has no inhibition for any antibiotics

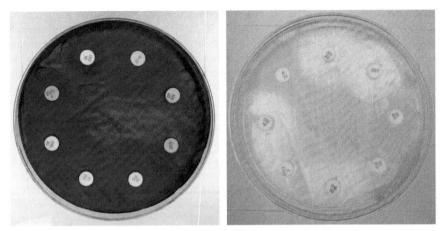

Fig. 6. Kirby Bauer disc diffusion method for antibiotic sensitivity. On the left is an example of a Mueller Hinton plate with 5% sheep blood with *Streptococcus zooepidemicus*. On the right is an example of a Mueller Hinton plate with *Escherichia coli*.

including large rafts of cells, intact individual cells, or disrupted UECs (see **Fig. 7**). Squamous epithelial cells are rare and usually only present in postpartum mares or mares refluxing urine into the uterus.[25–27] Squamous epithelial cells are typically evidence of cervical cell contamination. A large number of disrupted or degenerate uterine epithelial cells may indicate improper sample preparation, handling, or storage prior to staining or may be associated with a chronic uterine infection.

Debris Debris may be classified as none/minimal (<25% of the slide), mild (25%–50% of the slide), or moderate/severe (>75% of the slide). The presence of moderate-to-severe debris has been associated with bacterial endometritis. Additional diagnostic tests such as a low volume lavage may be indicated if a traditional uterine cytology sample shows moderate or severe debris with minimal evidence of inflammation (ie, a low number of WBCs).

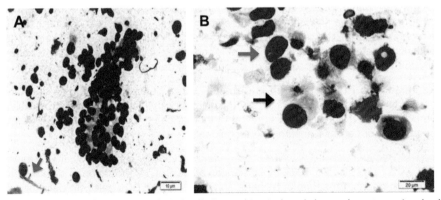

Fig. 7. (*A*) A raft of uterine epithelial cells (40× objective) and the nuclear streaming (*red arrow*). (*B*) individual ciliated UEC (*black arrow*) (100× oil objective), a UEC nucleus without cytoplasm (*red arrow*). (*From* Ferris RA, Bohn A, McCue PM. Equine endometrial cytology: collection techniques and interpretation. Equine Vet Educ 2015;27(6):316–22.)

White blood cells Neutrophils are the predominant WBC identified on uterine cytologic preparations (**Fig. 8**). Neutrophils are 10 to 12 μm in diameter (approximately twice as large as a red blood cell [RBC]), with a single nucleus that may be indented or divided into 3 to 5 lobes or segments. A cytology sample collected from a normal mare in estrus should have few or no neutrophils; occasionally a rare neutrophil may be noted associated with blood contamination during the collection process. Neutrophils will be present in the uterine lumen following breeding,[28] after uterine lavage[25] or infusion,[25] during the postpartum period,[25] or in cases of endometritis.

Other WBCs such as macrophages, lymphocytes, or eosinophils are not commonly found on equine uterine cytology preparations. Lymphocytes are approximately 7 μm in diameter (same size as an RBC), are round to oval, and have only a small amount of cytoplasm (see **Fig. 8**). Macrophages are approximately 20 μm in diameter with abundant blue staining cytoplasm filled with various sized vacuoles (see **Fig. 8**). Lymphocytes and macrophages are found in in the postpartum mare and in chronic uterine infections. Eosinophils are 12 to 15 μm in diameter, with blue staining cytoplasm that contains multiple pink or red granules (see **Fig. 8**). Eosinophils are found in cases of pneumovagina, fungal infections, or reflux of urine into the uterus.[26]

The average the number of white blood cells per hpf is determined after evaluating at least 10 hpf in multiple areas of the slide. The following categories may be used to define the presence/absence of white blood cells: normal (no WBC to rare WBC/hpf), mild inflammation (1–2 WBC/hpf), moderate inflammation (3–5 WBC/hpf) and severe inflammation (>5 WBC/hpf) (**Table 3**).[12,29,30] Another method used to categorize the inflammatory response is the number of WBCs per uterine epithelial cell. A ratio of 1 WBC to 20 to 40 epithelial cells has been used as a gauge of the degree of inflammation.[14,27] If the sample is of adequate cellularity, there is little to no difference between the 2 techniques in the ability to categorize the degree of inflammation. The number of WBCs per hpf does not apply to samples prepared from low volume lavage as epithelial cells and WBCs are concentrated during centrifugation. However, a ratio of WBC to UEC would still be appropriate.

Categorizing the degree of inflammation represented in a cytologic sample from a low volume lavage can be difficult. Centrifugation of the uterine effluent concentrates uterine epithelial cells, WBCs, microbial organisms, and debris into a pellet. The pellet is subsequently smeared onto a glass slide, stained, and evaluated. A normal mare should have few or no WBCs noted in the cytology from an low volume lavage (LVL). Mares with mild uterine inflammation often have more than 5 to 10 neutrophils per hpf, whereas mares with more severe inflammation usually have greater than 10 neutrophils per hpf. The presence of microbial organisms should be interpreted with caution, as there is a higher risk potential for contamination during sample collection with an LVL procedure versus use of a double-guarded uterine swab or brush.

Red blood cells RBCs are 6 μm in diameter with a central pallor. These cells are commonly found in low numbers (ie, <4/hpf) on routine cytologic evaluation. Excessive numbers of RBCs may indicate irritation to the endometrium from infection, infused compounds, or aggressive sampling technique.

Bacteria Bacteria can be visualized on a uterine cytology sample but often require 1000× (10× eye piece × 100× oil-immersion objective) magnification to differentiate them from debris. Presence of bacteria engulfed within WBCs can help determine if the bacteria are due to infectious endometritis or contamination. The 4 most common bacterial pathogens of the equine uterus are *Streptococcus equi* subspecies *zooepidemicus*, *E coli*, *Klebsiella pneumonia,* and *P aeruginosa. S equi* subspecies

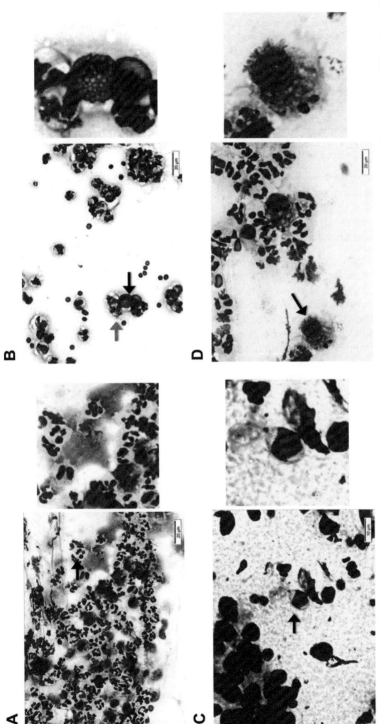

Fig. 8. WBCs from endometrial cytology samples. (*A*) UECs and numerous neutrophils (*black arrow*) and multiple neutrophils (*red arrow*) (100× oil objective). (*B*) An eosinophil (*black arrow*) and numerous neutrophils (*black arrow*) and numerous neutrophils (100× oil objective). (*D*) Multiple macrophages (*black arrow*) and neutrophils (100× oil objective; the area near the arrow is magnified on the right to allow for better visualization. (*From* Ferris RA, Bohn A, McCue PM. Equine endometrial cytology: collection techniques and interpretation. Equine Vet Educ 2015;27(6):316–22.)

Table 3
Description of the number of neutrophils per high power field with corresponding inflammation classification for samples collected from a brush/swab

Number of Neutrophils per hpf	Classification
0–Rare	Normal
1–2	Mild inflammation
3–5	Moderate inflammation
>5	Severe inflammation

From Ferris RA, Bohn A, McCue PM. Equine endometrial cytology: collection techniques and interpretation. Equine Vet Educ 2015;27(6);316–22.

zooepidemicus is a gram-positive cocci approximately 1.0 μm in diameter that forms chains of various length (**Fig. 9**). *E coli, K pneumonia, and P aeruginosa* are gram-negative rods varying in size from 3 to 6 μm in length and cannot be differentiated accurately based on cytologic evaluation.

Yeast/fungal organisms Yeasts are typically 5 to 8 μm in size with a distinct cell wall (100–200 nm) that forms a clear halo around the organism; this may be especially evident if the organism is surrounded by debris or other cells (see **Fig. 9**). Hyphate fungi are typically 3 to 5 μm in width and 8 μm in length. These individual cells are commonly linked together in long branching chains (see **Fig. 9**). In many instances, detection of a fungal organism on cytologic examination may be the only evidence of fungal endometritis, as organisms may not always grow on culture. If fungal organisms are detected, the microbiology laboratory should be notified so that the concurrent culture can be plate on media (ie, Sabouraud agar) to potentiate fungal growth.

The first step in interpretation of an endometrial cytology sample is determination if the sample is of adequate quality to be diagnostic. Subsequently, the sample is evaluated for evidence of inflammation and other abnormalities. The presence of more than 1 neutrophil per high power field from a traditional swab or brush cytology sample is an indication of inflammation, but does not necessarily indicate infection with a pathogenic organism. Typically, the number of neutrophils per hpf increases as the degree of inflammation increases within the uterus. In severe cases of endometritis, neutrophils may be so prevalent that few other cells can be identified.

Additional diagnostic tests

Molecular diagnostic tests are becoming common and replacing traditional bacterial and fungal cultivation in human and veterinary medicine.[31,32] These techniques are utilized when rapid identification or difficult-to-cultivate organisms are encountered. A quantitative polymerase chain reaction assay has been described for use in detecting fungal DNA within the uterine lumen due to the slow-growing nature of traditional fungal culture.[33] Currently, this technology is only available as a send-out diagnostic test; however, in human medicine, a platform is currently being utilized that allows for DNA amplification and detection to occur in a clinical setting in 1 to 2 hours. One of the limitations of this technology is that antibiotic sensitivity is not available with the results. In the future, whole-genome amplification of samples will allow for bacterial identification, prediction of antibiotic sensitivity, and presence of pathogenicity genes. This technology is currently being utilized in human medicine for the treatment of diabetic foot ulcers.[34]

Serum amyloid A (SAA) is an acute-phase protein that is upregulated in cases of bacterial infections in the horse.[35–41] Initial evaluations suggested that this acute-

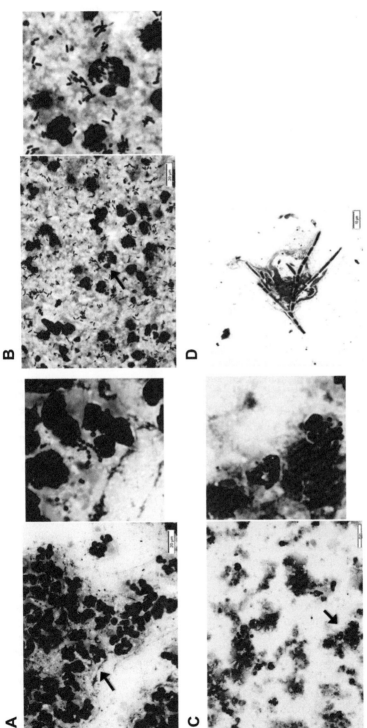

Fig. 9. Common pathogens found on endometrial cytology. (*A*) Neutrophils and cocci in chains (culture identified as *Streptococcus equi* subspecies *zooepidemicus*) (100× oil objective). (*B*) Neutrophils and rod-shaped bacteria (culture identified as *Escherichia coli*) (100× oil objective). (*C*) Neutrophils and yeast organisms (identified as *Candida albicans*) (100× oil objective). (*D*) Hyphate fungal organisms (identified as *Aspergillus fumigatus*) (100× oil objective). The panel on the left displays the image captured on 100× oil objective; the area near the arrow is magnified on the right to allow for better visualization. (*From* Ferris RA, Bohn A, McCue PM. Equine endometrial cytology: collection techniques and interpretation. Equine Vet Educ 2015;27(6):316–22.)

phase protein is upregulated systemically using a model of infectious endometritis.[37] However, larger clinical trials of naturally occurring cases of infectious endometritis do not support these findings.

Biofilm has been suggested to play a role in cases of chronic infectious endometritis.[2,42,43] It would be ideal to have a diagnostic marker to determine if cases of infectious endometritis involve a biofilm; however, currently there is not a marker for biofilm infections in human or veterinary medicine.[44,45] Recent work in the authors' laboratory has utilized screening methods to detect the bacterial specific signaling molecule cyclic-di-GMP that is only expressed when bacteria are living in a biofilm state. Currently, detection of cyclic-di-GMP is only available in specialized molecular core facilities. Future work is ongoing to identify a rapid method of detecting cyclic-di-GMP as a marker of biofilm associated infections.

Hysteroscopy can be utilized to visualize the endometrial surface for abnormalities. It has been suggested that in cases of chronic endometritis individual sporadic adherent plaques of bacterial and fungal pathogens can be detected.[2] A culture instrument can be either passed next to or through the endoscope to collect a guided sample from the plaque for microbial culture and cytologic evaluation as described in this article.

SUMMARY

Detection of infectious endometritis, while challenging in certain cases, usually can be easily diagnosed or ruled out using a sample from a guarded swab and cytology brush, small volume lavage, or uterine biopsy. These samples are routinely submitted for microbial culture and cytologic evaluation. However, there is not a gold standard diagnostic sample or analysis of the sample that is quick to perform, is inexpensive, and returns rapid results.

In a clinical setting, an option for screening mares with infectious endometritis is to use a guarded culture swab and cytology brush for microbial culture and cytologic evaluation. If the results are positive, the causative organism and antibiotic susceptibility can be determined to generate an appropriate therapeutic plan. If the results are negative for infectious endometritis but the mare has several risk factors or clinical signs (eg, intrauterine fluid, or cervical discharge), further diagnostics are warranted such as a small volume lavage or uterine biopsy to confirm or rule out infectious endometritis.

REFERENCES

1. Traub-Dargatz JL, Salman MD, Voss JL. Medical problems of adult horses, as ranked by equine practitioners. J Am Vet Med Assoc 1991;198(10):1745–7.
2. LeBlanc MM, Causey RC. Clinical and subclinical endometritis in the mare: both threats to fertility. Reprod Domest Anim 2009;44(Suppl 3):10–22.
3. Burleson MD, LeBlanc MM, Riddle WT. Endometrial microbial isolates are associated with different ultrasonographic and endometrial cytology findings in Thoroughbred mares. Proc Am Assoc Eq Pract 2010;56:317.
4. Bohn AA, Ferris RA, McCue PM. Comparison of equine endometrial cytology samples collected with uterine swab, uterine brush, and low-volume lavage from healthy mares. Vet Clin Pathol 2014;43(4):594–600.
5. Overbeck W, Witte TS, Heuwieser W. Comparison of three diagnostic methods to identify subclinical endometritis in mares. Theriogenology 2011;75(7):1311–8.
6. Defontis M, Vaillancourt D, Grand FX. Comparison of three methods of sampling for endometrial cytology in the mare. Tierarztl Prax Ausg G Grosstiere Nutztiere 2011;39(3):171–5.

7. Aguilar J, Hanks M, Shaw DJ, et al. Importance of using guarded techniques for the preparation of endometrial cytology smears in mares. Theriogenology 2006; 66(2):423–30.

8. Wingfield Digby NJ, Ricketts SW. Results of concurrent bacteriological and cytological examinations of the endometrium of mares in routine stud farm practice 1978-1981. J Reprod Fertil Suppl 1982;32:181–5.

9. Ricketts SW. Microbiological culture techniques and interpretation. In Equine Reproduction, 2nd edition. McKinnon AO, Squires EL, Valla WE, et al, editors. Vol. 2, Chapter 208. Wiley Blackwell; 2011. p. 1963–78.

10. Ricketts SW, Mackintosh ME. Role of anaerobic bacteria in equine endometritis. J Reprod Fertil Suppl 1987;35:343–51.

11. Nielsen JM. Endometritis in the mare: a diagnostic study comparing cultures from swab and biopsy. Theriogenology 2005;64(3):510–8.

12. Riddle WT, LeBlanc MM, Stromberg AJ. Relationships between uterine culture, cytology and pregnancy rates in a Thoroughbred practice. Theriogenology 2007;68(3):395–402.

13. Nielsen JM, Troedsson MH, Pedersen MR, et al. Diagnosis of endometritis in the mare based on bacteriological and cytological examinations of the endometrium: comparison of results obtained by swabs and biopsies. J Equine Vet Sci 2010; 30(1):27–30.

14. Ball BA, Shin SJ, Patten VH, et al. Use of a low-volume uterine flush for microbiologic and cytologic examination of the mare's endometrium. Theriogenology 1988;29(6):1269–83.

15. LeBlanc MM, Magsig J, Stromberg AJ. Use of a low-volume uterine flush for diagnosing endometritis in chronically infertile mares. Theriogenology 2007;68(3): 403–12.

16. Cocchia N, Paciello O, Auletta L, et al. Comparison of the cytobrush, cottonswab, and low volume uterine flush techniques to evaluate endometrial cytology for diagnosing endometritis in chronically infertile mares. Theriogenology 2012;77:89–98.

17. Kenney RM. Prognostic value of endometrial biopsy of the mare. J Reprod Fertil Suppl 1975;23:347–8.

18. Doig PA, McKnight JD, Miller RB. The use of endometrial biopsy in the infertile mare. Can Vet J 1981;22(3):72–6.

19. Ricketts SW, Alonso S. Assessment of the breeding prognosis of mares using paired endometrial biopsy techniques. Equine Vet J 1991;23(3):185–8.

20. Nielsen JM, Nielsen FH, Petersen MR. Diagnosis of equine endometritis - Microbiology, cytology and histology of endometrial biopsies and the correlation to fertility. Pferdeheilkunde 2012;28:8–13.

21. Hartman DL, Bliss S. Laboratory Methods for isolation and evaluation of bacteira, fungi, and yeasts. In: McKinnon AO, Squires EL, Vaala WE, et al, editors. Equine reproduction. West sussex (United Kingdom): Wiley-Blackwell; 2011. p. 2674–81.

22. Beehan DP, McKinnon AO. How to diagnose common equine reproductive tract bacterial pathognes using chromogenic agar. Proc Am Assoc Eq Pract 2009;55: 320–5.

23. Dascanio JJ, Schweizer C, Ley WB. Equine fungal endometritis. Equine Vet 2001; 13(6):324–9.

24. Roszel JF, Freeman KP. Equine endometrial cytology. Vet Clin N Am-equine Pract 1988;4(2):247–62.

25. Saltiel A, Gutierrez A, de Buen-Llado N, et al. Cervico-endometrial cytology and physiological aspects of the post-partum mare. J Reprod Fertil Suppl 1987;35: 305–9.

26. Slusher SH, Freeman KP, Roszel JF. Eosinophils in equine uterine cytology and histology specimens. J Am Vet Med Assoc 1984;184(6):665–70.
27. Couto MA, Hughes JP. Technique and interpretation of cervical and endometrial cytology in the mare. J Equine Vet Sci 1984;4(6):265–73.
28. Card C. Post-breeding inflammation and endometrial cytology in mares. Theriogenology 2005;64(3):580–8.
29. Brook D. Uterine culture in mares. Mod Vet Pract 1984;65(5):A3–8.
30. Knudsen O. Endometrial cytology as a diagnostic aid in mares. Cornell Vet 1964; 54:415–22.
31. Fischer N, Indenbirken D, Meyer T, et al. Evaluation of Unbiased Next-Generation Sequencing of RNA (RNA-seq) as a Diagnostic Method in Influenza Virus-Positive Respiratory Samples. J Clin Microbiol 2015;53:2238–50.
32. Halliday CL, Kidd SE, Sorrell TC, et al. Molecular diagnostic methods for invasive fungal disease: the horizon draws nearer? Pathology 2015;47:257–69.
33. Ferris RA, Dern K, Veir JK, et al. Development of a broad-range quantitative polymerase chain reaction assay to detect and identify fungal DNA in equine endometrial samples. Am J Vet Res 2013;74:161–5.
34. Lavigne J-P, Sotto A, Dunyach-Remy C, et al. New Molecular Techniques to Study the Skin Microbiota of Diabetic Foot Ulcers. Adv Wound Care 2015;4:38–49.
35. da Silva MC, Canisso IF. Serum amyloid A concentration in healthy periparturient mares and mares with ascending placentitis. Equine Vet J 2013;45:619–24.
36. Canisso IF, Ball BA, Cray C, et al. Use of a qualitative horse-side test to measure serum amyloid a in mares with experimentally induced ascending placentitis. J Equine Vet Sci 2015;35:54–9.
37. Mette C, Camilla Dooleweerdt B, Stine J, et al. Evaluation of the systemic acute phase response and endometrial gene expression of serum amyloid A and pro- and anti-inflammatory cytokines in mares with experimentally induced endometritis. Vet Immunol Immunopathol 2010;138:95–105.
38. Belgrave RL, Dickey MM, Arheart KL, et al. Assessment of serum amyloid A testing of horses and its clinical application in a specialized equine practice. J Am Vet Med Assoc 2013;243:113–9.
39. Jacobsen S, Thomsen MH, Nanni S. Concentrations of serum amyloid A in serum and synovial fluid from healthy horses and horses with joint disease. Am J Vet Res 2006;67:1738–42.
40. Jacobsen S, Andersen PH. The acute phase protein serum amyloid A (SAA) as a marker of inflammation in horses. Equine Vet Educ 2007;19:38–46.
41. Hulten C, Demmers S. Serum amyloid A (SAA) as an aid in the management of infectious disease in the foal: comparison with total leucocyte count, neutrophil count and fibrinogen. Equine Vet J 2002;34:693–8.
42. Ferris RA, McCue PM, Borlee GI, et al. In vitro efficacy of nonantibiotic treatments on biofilm disruption of gram-negative pathogens and an in vivo model of infectious endometritis utilizing isolates from the equine uterus. J Clin Microbiol 2016; 54:631–9.
43. Beehan DP, Wolfsdorf K, Elam J, et al. The evaluation of biofilm-forming potential of Escherichia coli collected from the equine female reproductive tract. J Equine Vet Sci 2015;35:935–9.
44. Donlan RM. Biofilm elimination on intravascular catheters: important considerations for the infectious disease practitioner. Clin Infect Dis 2011;52:1038–45.
45. Clutterbuck AL, Woods EJ, Knottenbelt DC, et al. Biofilms and their relevance to veterinary medicine. Vet Microbiol 2007;121:1–17.

Endometritis

Nontraditional Therapies

Charles F. Scoggin, DVM, MS

KEYWORDS

- Subfertility • Broodmare • Pregnancy • Endometritis

KEY POINTS

- Traditional therapies for endometritis comprise the use of intrauterine and systemic antimicrobial agents, uterine lavage, and ecbolic agent.
- Alternative therapies are those using medications or devices in an off-label manner.
- These therapies are used when traditional therapies fail or are no longer viable.

INTRODUCTION

Myriad options, opinions, and even dogmas exist for the treatment of endometritis in the mare. Indications for and success rates of these treatments are variably represented in research abstracts, clinical reports, and anecdotal observations. Traditional therapies typically consist of systemic or intrauterine (IU) antibiotics, uterine irrigation, and ecbolics. These can be used in tandem and often prove successful in management of endometritis in most cases. For more thorough descriptions of traditional therapies, the reader is directed to current reviews pertaining to management of the subfertile mare.

However, there are some cases when either traditional therapies fall short or the problem recrudesces. In these instances, nontraditional or alternative therapies may be pursued either as adjunctive or stand-alone measures. A variable body of evidenced-based data exists for many of these treatments. There is also a healthy dose of anecdotal reports that spur the use of many of these modalities. Difficulty

Disclosure/Conflicts of Interest: The author is employed by an equine hospital that is directly affiliated with a veterinary pharmacy. Many of the pharmaceuticals discussed here can be purchased from this and other veterinary pharmacies and distributors. In addition, some treatments listed here have only anecdotal evidence to support their use and/or require the use of compounded medications. Readers are thus cautioned to use the treatments and medications appropriately, judiciously, and ethically. No guarantee and warrantee can be made regarding the efficacy of these treatments; use is at the sole discretion of the clinician administering the medications.
LeBlanc Reproduction Center, Rood and Riddle Equine Hospital, 2150 Georgetown Road, Lexington, KY 40511, USA
E-mail address: cscoggin@roodandriddle.com

thus arises when attempting to define or corral the term "alternative." Such a term is associated with a certain level of mysticism and, at its extremes, may represent generalized quackery by being in direct opposition to Western medicine theories and practices. None of the treatments discussed here fall into that latter category. Instead, the terms "alternative" or "nontraditional" (or other equivalents) are used to refer to treatments considered medical devices or medications used in an off-label manner.[1] The author warns readers that liberty is taken with this definition when discussing certain treatments; nevertheless, all therapies are accompanied by some credible evidence for their use.

Regardless of the treatment, all theriogenologists would agree that no matter how innovative the approach, it is for naught if the underlying causes are not properly identified. It thus behooves the clinician to be thorough and, in some instances, leave no stone unturned before investing in treatment. Methods used to diagnose endometritis are beyond the scope of this article and are discussed elsewhere.[2] Instead, this discussion reviews traditional and alternative therapies used in cases of endometritis.

PATIENT EVALUATION OVERVIEW

Inflammation of the uterus following breeding is considered a normal yet transient physiologic response.[3] Current estimates suggest that 80% to 90% of mares are capable of managing this inflammation with little to no intervention; these individuals are considered reproductively normal or resistant mares. The other 10% to 20% either has or is prone to some type of endometritis and are considered susceptible mares. Causes for susceptibility include:

- Age and parity
- Colonization of the reproductive tract with pathogenic organisms
- Chronic degenerative endometritis
- Anatomic and functional defects
- Aberrant local immune response
- Method of breeding

These causes are not mutually exclusive and can work in tandem to adversely affect mares' reproductive efficiency. Treatment is based on identifying and addressing the sources for the inflammation and/or contamination. Once identified, the clinician can devise and implement a therapeutic plan to maximize the mare's fertility.

Biofilm Infections

Biofilm is a hot topic in equine reproduction and deserves its own section for discussion. As a review, bacteria can exist in one of two states. The first is the free-floating or planktonic state; the second is the biofilm state produced by a community of bacteria. Biofilm is thought to provide an added barrier of protection against the host's immune system and antibiotic agents, thereby causing persistent infections. Research investigating the actual presence of biofilm within the mare's uterus is currently underway, and an experimental model has proven promising in studying this phenomenon.[4] Nevertheless, there are clinical accounts and anecdotal reports of successful treatment of presumed biofilm infections.[5,6] Various pathogenic bacteria have been implicated in biofilm formation, including *Escherichia coli*, *Klebsiella pneumoniae*, *Pseudomonas aeruginosa*, and *Streptococcus equi* ssp *zooepidemicus*. Research is ongoing studying the efficacy of certain agents for combatting biofilm infections in broodmares.

PHARMACOLOGIC TREATMENT OPTIONS
Antibacterial Agents

Antibacterial agents have been used in broodmare reproduction for decades as a means of prophylaxis or therapy for infectious endometritis. However, antibacterial agents are not benign. IU treatments during diestrus can predispose mares to fungal endometritis,[7] systemic therapy may disrupt gastrointestinal flora and lead to enterocolitis,[8] and the firestorm of antimicrobial resistance is posing a global health threat.[9] Consequently, selection of a suitable antibacterial agent should ideally be based on culture and sensitivity, and any other health issues or past medical history. Route of administration (eg, systemic vs IU) should be chosen with consideration to the stage of the mare's estrous cycle. Combination therapy can also be performed and is often done so with good clinical results.

Systemic and Intrauterine Antibacterial Drugs

Table 1 lists common drug dosages used in broodmare reproduction to treat infectious endometritis. Considerations for the use of systemic antibacterial agents include culture and sensitivity results, ability to achieve effective concentrations in the urogenital system, practicality and availability of drug administration, and compatibility with other medications. Advantages of systemic antibacterials are

- Ability to treat irrespective of the stage of the estrous cycle
- Maintenance of steady therapeutic concentrations for a prolonged period of time
- Less susceptible to an adverse intraluminal uterine environment
- Eliminates risk of iatrogenic contamination of the reproductive tract

One major disadvantage of systemic treatment is increased cost in terms of drug volume and veterinary services required. Other disadvantages were previously discussed.

IU antibiotics are another option and are likely more commonly used than systemic drugs.[10,11] Considerations for use are strikingly different. First, use of IU infusions during diestrus may increase the risk of fungal endometritis.[7] Although this concern is justified, the risk is abated with careful patient selection and administration of a luteolytic dose of prostaglandin $F_{2\alpha}$ (PGF$_{2\alpha}$) to lyse the corpus luteum (CL), relax the cervix, and promote uterine clearance. Other important considerations are that it remains relatively nonirritating to the endometrium and/or external genitalia, it maintains stability when mixed with another agent or solution, it achieves appropriate mean inhibitory concentrations for the pathogens of interest, and it has a specific effect on bacterial metabolism. One of the most commonly used antibiotics for IU infusion (ticarcillin + clavulonic acid) seems to require twice-daily infusions to maintain appropriate mean inhibitory concentrations against β-streptococci.[11,12] Conversely, treatment with ceftiofur, another widely used antibacterial drug, needs only once-daily infusions.[13] A recent collaborative report from Washington State University and clinicians in Kentucky reported on the relative efficacy of a water-based 2.5% enrofloxacin solution.[14] Such a treatment can prove useful in combating susceptible infections and seems to be much safer than when using the commercial preparation of enrofloxacin available for systemic use.

Whether using systemic or IU antibacterial agents, empirical therapy may be considered or even necessary when a delay in treatment can have negative consequences. Studies comparing the effects of systemic versus IU or other therapies are lacking. However, clinical experience suggests that systemic therapy is a useful part of treating mares with acute and chronic endometritis. Nevertheless, such a

Table 1
Dosages for common antibacterial agents used in equine reproduction

Medication	Systemic Dosage	Intra-uterine Dosage	Indications/Comments
Amikacin	10–15 mg/kg, IV, q 24 h	1–2 g, q 24 h	Buffer with equal parts 8.4% sodium bicarbonate and qs to ≥60 mL with sterile saline when giving IU
Ampicillin sodium	29 mg/kg, IV or IM, q 12 h	2 g, q 24 h	qs to ≥60 mL with sterile saline when giving IU; may precipitate in uterus and cause irritation
Ceftiofur sodium	2 mg/kg, IV or IM, q 12–24 h	1–2 g, q 24 h	qs to ≥60 mL with sterile saline when giving IU
Ceftiofur sodium crystalline free acid	6.6 mg/kg, IM, 2 doses 4 d apart	Not studied or recommended at this time	Will reach therapeutic concentrations within endometrium
Enrofloxacin	5–7.5 mg/kg, IV, q 24 h; 7.5 mg/kg, PO, q 12 h	50 mL of water-based 2.5% suspension,[a] q 24 h	Do NOT use commercial preparation IU
Gentamicin	6.6 mg/kg, IV or IM, q 24 h	1–2 g, q 24 h	Buffer with equal parts 8.4% sodium bicarbonate and qs to ≥60 mL with sterile saline when giving IU
Polymixin B	5000 U/kg, IV, q 8–12 h	1,000,000 U OR 1 million units, q 24 h	Dilute in at least 1 L fluids when giving IV; qs to ≥60 mL with sterile saline when giving IU
Potassium penicillin G	20,000–40,000 U, IV, q 6 h	5 million units, q 12–24 h	qs to at least 35 mL with sterile water or saline when giving IU
Procaine penicillin G	20,000–40,000 U, IM, q 12 h	5 million units, q 12–24 h	qs to ≥35 mL with sterile water or saline when giving IU
Ticarcillin + clavulonic acid	50 mg/kg, IV or IM, q 6–8 h	3.1–6.2 g, q 12–24 h	qs to ≥60 mL with sterile saline when giving IU

Abbreviations: IM, intramuscularly; IV, intravenously.
  [a] Requires compounding.

statement should not be confused with the widespread or "treat 'em all" approach. With concerns about antimicrobial resistance reaching near pandemic levels, this practice is no longer condoned. A more prudent and scrupulous course of action is to use antimicrobial agents when there is solid clinical and/or diagnostic evidence for treatment. Indeed, a recent review[15] regarding the prophylactic use of IU antibiotics concluded that despite justifiable pressures, use of antimicrobials in this manner was highly questionable and recommended early intervention with ecbolics and uterine irrigation (discussed next).

Ecbolic Agents

The value of ecbolic agents has been known for some time.[16] Oxytocin is a neuropeptide produced in the hypothalamus and released by the posterior pituitary. It is frequently given exogenously to promote myometrial contractions and thus clearance of fluid and debris from the uterus. Consideration should be given to stage of estrous cycle when giving oxytocin. Intravenous administration of 30 units to estrus mares was shown to reduce uterine contractions compared with lower doses of 5 to 10 units.[17] The density of oxytocin receptors is highest in late diestrus and decreases during estrus and early diestrus,[18] and the uterine response to oxytocin is inversely related to progesterone concentrations.[19] Recommended doses are 10 to 20 units during estrus and 25 to 40 units after ovulation to achieve the desired effect.[2] Routes of administration include intravenous, intramuscular, and IU. Oxytocin is by no means a "silver bullet" and its effects are limited by anatomic (eg, closed cervix and pendulous uterus) and mechanical (eg, fibrosis leading to aberrant contractions) deficits concurrently involving the reproductive tract. A synthetic analogue, carbetocin, has been available in countries outside the United States. Its plasma half-life is more than two-times that of oxytocin and may be useful in mares that do not respond to oxytocin.[20]

Oxytocin is directly responsible for release of prostaglandins from the endometrium. $PGF_{2\alpha}$ is the primary prostaglandin released by the endometrium to remove or lyse the CL. In addition to its luteolytic effect, it is also a useful ecbolic agent. Treatment with 250 μg of cloprostenol, a synthetic analogue of $PGF_{2\alpha}$, produces the best response among the $PGF_{2\alpha}$ preparations studied.[21] When comparing the ecbolic effects of oxytocin and $PGF_{2\alpha}$, the former produces strong and rapid uterine contractions over a relatively short period of time ($\sim$30 minutes). The latter produces lower-amplitude contractions over a longer time period (4–6 hours). These varying effects are taken into consideration when implementing treatment. Attention should be paid to timing of $PGF_{2\alpha}$ treatment. Some evidence exists that treatment during early diestrus may impair CL function, although it does not seem to affect fertility.[22]

Other drugs potentially affecting uterine contractility are the α_2-agonist sedatives and nonsteroidal anti-inflammatory drugs. Detomidine causes contractions in normal mares,[23] whereas nonsteroidal anti-inflammatory drugs, because of their inhibitory action on inducible prostaglandin release, may inhibit uterine clearance and/or cause ovulation failure.[24]

Uterine Irrigation/Lavage

Uterine irrigation or lavage is a useful tool in the breeding management of problem or susceptible mares. This technique follows the timeless dictum of "the solution to pollution is dilution." Consequently, the goal of uterine lavage is to assist with clearance of inflammatory debris within the uterus. Lavage with lactated Ringer solution (LRS) immediately before insemination or mating does not adversely affect pregnancy rates[25] and likely does not interfere with sperm function or passage to the uterine tubes (site of fertilization).[26] Lavage should be withheld until approximately 4 hours after breeding.[27] Fluid choice is somewhat clinician dependent, but most theriogenologists prefer a balanced polyionic fluid, such as LRS. Saline (0.9%) may also be used. Volume and frequency is contingent on the severity of endometritis. Breeding management typically relies on 2 to 4 L once or twice a day. Additives are commonly mixed into lavage fluids in a multimodal approach to therapy (discussed later).

ALTERNATIVE TREATMENT OPTIONS

The previously mentioned therapies are mainstays of treatment of endometritis. However, they are not the only options for therapy, with almost countless treatments described in the literature and discussed anecdotally. Reviewing all options available is a daunting task, yet doing so allows for a comparison of these different modalities, some of which are provided in **Table 2**. What follows is a discussion of various alternative treatments for endometritis, including their indications and limitations.

Antimicrobial Peptides

Antimicrobial peptides are produced and used by neutrophils to degrade bacteria. Purportedly, antimicrobial peptides need only come in contact with bacteria cell membranes to exert a bactericidal effect. Other attributes include a broad-spectrum of activity, less risk of developing resistance to microbial defense mechanisms, and direct activity against biofilm. Ceragyn is a commercially available wound-healing medical device marketed as an antimicrobial peptide mimic. In vitro studies evaluating its activity against clinical isolates of common urogenital pathogens have been promising. Ceragyn was effective in killing free-floating and biofilm-protected isolates of *S equi* ssp *zooepidemicus*, *E coli*, and *K pneumoniae* in all samples studied.[28] Its efficacy against *P aeruginosa* in a free-floating state was also deemed good, but it was inconsistent in disrupting this particular bacterium in a biofilm state. These researchers also

Table 2
Nontraditional therapeutics for treatment of endometritis

Intrauterine Therapies			
Agent	Dose/Volume	Frequency	Indications
Ceragyn	60 mL/2 oz (1 vial)	>4 h before breeding or 6–48 h after breeding	IE, PMIE, and suspect biofilm infection
Hydrogen peroxide (3% U.S.P.)	20 mL qs to 60 mL w/LRS 100 mL in 1 L LRS	6–48 h after breeding or concurrently with an infusion of an antimicrobial	IE, PMIE, and suspect biofilm infection
Acetylcysteine (20% solution)	30 mL in 150–250 mL saline	24–48 h before breeding and 24 h before infusion of an antimicrobial	IE, PMIE, and suspect biofilm infection
Tricide (EDTA-Tris)	250–500 mL	Synergistic effect and can be given with aminoglycocides and clotrimazole	IE and suspect biofilm production
Kerosene	500 mL	Once; lavage 12–24 h after infusion	CDE
Plasma (autologous)	90 mL[a]	Once; 12–36 h after breeding	PMIE
Platelet-rich plasma	10 mL[b]	Once; 24–35 h before breeding	PMIE
Mesenchymal stem cells, allogenic	20×10^6 qs to 20 mL with LRS[c]	24 h before breeding	PMIE
Autologous conditioned serum	20 mL[c]	24 h before breeding	PMIE
bActivate	10 mL	24 h before culture	IE (subclinical)

Abbreviations: CDE, chronic degenerative endometritis; IE, infectious endometritis; PMIE, persistent-mating-induced endometritis.
[a] Can be given in combination with penicillin and neomycin as reported by Pascoe.[43]
[b] Platelet-rich plasma harvesting system was the Angel Cytomedix, Inc (Gaithersburg, MD) and resulting yield was qs to 10 mL with platelet-poor plasma as reported by Metcalf and coworkers.[44]
[c] As reported by Ferris and coworkers.[46]

noted that Ceragyn's greatest efficacy (or killing power) occurred between 6 and 12 hours after infusion.

Ceragyn is labeled for use 4 hours before or 6 to 48 hours after breeding. It is most commonly used as a uterine infusion that is deposited and left in the uterus. This product is also labeled as a lavage device for in-and-out uterine irrigation. Additionally, Ceragyn is used to treat active cases of endometritis, whereby it is infused following uterine culture, cytology, and biopsy as an empirical therapy. The following day, uterine lavage is performed and treatment can be repeated or followed with infusion of an appropriate antibacterial agent. Anecdotal reports from practitioners in the field using Ceragyn have been favorable if not enthusiastic.

Immunomodulators

Influencing either systemic or local immune defense systems in the management of endometritis has been investigated in broodmares. Corticosteroids have been used to manage susceptible mares to reduce neutrophil margination into the uterus, and a treatment of lymphangectasia. The clinical benefit of a dexamethasone was described by Bucca and colleagues in which they reported improved pregnancy rates in susceptible mares treated with 50 mg (intramuscularly) of dexamethasone before breeding.[28] Prednisolone (0.1 mg/kg, twice a day by mouth) beginning 2 days before breeding has also been used to manage acute inflammation when breeding with frozen semen.[29] When using corticosteroids, patient selection is important because of potential untoward side effects of steroid administration in equids, such as laminitis and muscle wasting.

Upregulation of local defense mechanisms has been explored as a means to improve fertility rates in susceptible mares. More specifically, improving the phagocytic activity of mononuclear cells and reducing the production of proinflammatory cytokines are possible benefits of altering uterine immune systems. Mares treated with a commercially available *Mycobacterium* cell-wall extract showed a significant reduction in inflammation compared with control animals.[30] A similar product containing *Proprionibacterium acnes* was shown to increase pregnancy and live-foal rates in barren mares treated with this product and conventional management strategies.[31] Use of these agents for endometritis thus seems to warrant more consideration in the management of endometritis, especially persistent-mating-induced endometritis (PMIE).

Some researchers postulate that certain bacteria can exist in a dormant stage within the uterus and may be an important cause of subclinical endometritis in broodmares.[32,33] In the dormant phase, bacteria are not actively dividing and propagating; instead, they are metabolically inactive, allowing them to evade local immune defense mechanisms and common antibacterial agents. Reactivation of these bacteria with a proprietary medical device (bActivate, Hagyard Veterinary Pharmacy, Lexington, KY) has been proposed to diagnose and treat subfertile mares in instances where a chronic infection with *S equi* ssp *equi* (β-*Strep*) is suspected, but standard culture and cytology yield equivocal results.[34] A field study performed in Central Kentucky reported improved pregnancy and live-foal rates when this product was used in the management of barren mares.[32,33] In addition, researchers reported a 64% reactivation rate (ie, subjects that originally cultured negative but cultured positive for β-*Strep* 24 hours after bActivate was infused) in mares when bActivate was used as an aid in management of these mares. This product is available for purchase in the United States from a veterinary pharmacy.

Hydrogen Peroxide

Long-used as an antiseptic, H_2O_2 has a broad-spectrum of activity against various microbes, including bacteria, virus, fungi, yeast, and spores. In mares, the recommended dose is 20 mL of a 3% solution diluted to 60 mL in LRS.[35] An in vitro study demonstrated that 1% H_2O_2 is useful against most pathogens in their planktonic and biofilm state, except for P aeruginosa, which was capable of inactivating H_2O_2.[36] The mode of action is disruption of the cellular membrane and intracellular DNA. Contact time with H_2O_2 seems to be key because it is rapidly degraded by catalase, which is found in many tissue systems.[37] Irrigation with dilute H_2O_2 (100 mL of 3% H_2O_2) has been used by some clinicians in cases of known β-Strep infections. This obviously represents a significant dilution but has provided good clinical results. Clinically, there is minimal inflammatory response following either infusion or lavage with H_2O_2. Bacterial resistance to H_2O_2 has been documented in human cases but research is lacking in horses.

N-Acetylcysteine

This agent has been used as a mucolytic to treat respiratory conditions and as part of retention enemas for meconium impactions. Clinical studies in the mid-2000s indicated that N-acetylcysteine can be used successfully to treat subfertile mares.[5] Mares treated with N-acetylcysteine before breeding had higher fertility rates than those that were not, and treatment had no adverse effects on the endometrium as judged by uterine biopsy. Proposed mechanisms of action include reduction in viscosity of mucus within the endometrium and anti-inflammatory properties.[38,39] Treatment involves diluting a 20% (200 mg/mL) solution in 150 mL to 250 mL of saline and instilling it into the uterus. This is done 24 to 48 before or 6 to 24 hours after breeding. Serial uterine lavages are often performed 12 to 24 hours after infusion and repeated until the efflux is clear. Instillation of N-acetylcysteine is a good empirical treatment and avoids the indiscriminate use of antibiotics. Although long-term clinical success is based on pregnancy rates, short-term effects are often realized by retrieval of mucoid and tenacious effluent.

Chelating Agents

Chelating agents offer an intriguing treatment option in cases of refractory bacterial and fungal infections. Use of 8-mM disodium EDTA dehydrate and 20-mM 2-amino-2-hydroxymethyl-1, 3-propanediol (Tricide, Rood and Riddle Veterinary Pharmacy, Lexington, KY) has been shown to potentiate the effects of certain antimicrobial agents by lowering their respective mean-inhibitory concentrations.[40] The mechanism of action is proposed to be via altering cell-wall permeability.[39] Between 250 mL and 500 mL of Tricide are infused into the uterus on the first day of treatment, followed by uterine irrigation 12 to 24 hours later. Subsequent infusions can be performed, and concurrent treatment with intrauterine antibiotics is possible. Aminoglycosides are reported to have a synergistic effect with Tricide, and the two can be mixed together without any precipitate forming. Note that β-lactam antibiotics can precipitate in the presence of Tricide, which may inactivate these antibiotics. When treating with known culture and sensitivity results, the author's preference is to add 2 g of gentamicin sulfate to Tricide just before instillation. Uterine irrigation and additional infusions can be performed daily. In vitro studies evaluating the use of a similar chelating agent, tris-EDTA, showed it to be highly effective on E coli in a planktonic state but inconsistent in reducing the number of colony-forming units and disrupting biofilm production from clinical isolates of P aeruginosa or K pneumonia.[4] Based on these data, it seems that Tricide and other chelating agents should be reserved for confirmed E coli infections.

Kerosene

Kerosene is a clear liquid formed by fractional distillation of petroleum. Used for more than 100 years as a fuel, it is also a useful solvent for removing grease and tenacious mucilage, and as a pesticide for killing lice and bed bugs. The use of kerosene as a treatment of subfertile mares was first reported by Bracher and colleagues.[41] Researchers reported high early pregnancy (87.5%) rates in mares treated with kerosene on the cycle before mating. However, live-foal rates were mediocre at best (62.5%). Despite inducing an intense and, in some cases, diphtheroid inflammation, no long-term side effects (eg, cervical or uterine adhesions) were observed in the mares treated with kerosene. In addition, anecdotal and clinical experience indicates that kerosene can be used at any stage of the estrous cycle, including diestrus and 48 hours before breeding.

Mares who have gone more than 1 year barren, have not responded favorably following multiple cycles of IU therapies, or have severe IU fluid accumulation are candidates for uterine infusion of kerosene. Treatment is thought to perform a chemical curettage of the endometrial epithelium,[42] effectively stripping the endothelium of debris, inspissated material, and microorganisms, thereby providing a more hospitable environment for a developing embryo. Treatment protocols vary primarily by volume used, with infusions ranging from 90 mL to 500 mL, followed by uterine lavage the next day (and successive days if indicated). Effluent character ranges from mostly clear (yet strongly odorous of kerosene) to mucoid to hemorrhagic with the consistency of curdled milk.

The author's technique is similar to that described by Bracher and colleagues,[41] but there were a few notable exceptions. Briefly, kerosene is obtained from a commercial source (eg, gas station) and placed in a clean, nonflammable plastic container. Mares are prepared routinely for a vaginal procedure with careful cleansing of the vulva with moist cotton and 2% chlorhexidine scrub. A sterile palpation sleeve is donned and a new, clean Harris flush tube (24F catheter, 60-inch length) is grasped, and the tip fed through the external os of the cervix until entering the lumen of the uterus. A plastic receptacle (eg, clean funnel or large catheter syringe without the plunger) is attached to the other end of the tube. Approximately 250 mL to 500 mL of kerosene is poured into the receptacle by an assistant and allowed to flow by gravity through the tube and into the uterus. Once the entire volume is deposited within the uterine lumen, the tube is removed, and the cervix held close for 5 to 10 seconds to prevent reflux of the fluid. Because of the flammable nature of kerosene, mares are usually placed in an outdoor paddock as soon as the infusions are complete because of concern about leaking kerosene in the stall and bedding, which could pose a fire hazard. All disposable items are double-bagged and discarded in a dumpster. Approximately 16 to 24 hours after infusion, the uterus is irrigated with physiologic saline or LRS until the effluent is clear. Uterine irrigation is repeated daily as necessary, and mares are managed routinely for live-cover matings or artificial insemination. The author and another clinician recently reviewed records from 25 mares under their care in which this protocol was used in subfertile mares that had been barren for at least 2 years. Fifteen (60%) of these mares became pregnant, as judged by either 8-day embryo recovery rates or 14-day pregnancy examinations, within two cycles after therapy (Cook and Scoggin, unpublished data, 2015). To date, live-foal rates and statistical analyses have not been evaluated, so these results should be interpreted with caution.

The author recognizes that IU treatment with kerosene is considered taboo, if not unkind, by some of his peers. Moreover, its use also has the perception as a stop-gap procedure used only after all else has failed. However, when used appropriately and judiciously, it can yield positive results. Because of its properties as a solvent, the author has found this treatment highly beneficial in cases of confirmed (as evidenced by endometrial biopsy) cystic glandular distention and inspissation. Unfortunately, whether or not these effects are truly realized has not been confirmed by the author because follow-up biopsies are seldom pursued after treatment.

Regenerative Therapies

The use of autologous and allogenic biologics, also referred to as regenerative therapies, has been explored for their efficacy in the management of endometritis. Higher pregnancy rates were reported in lactating mares when treated with an IU infusion of autologous plasma and antibiotics compared with control mares.[43] Clinical reports of allogenic plasma (eg, frozen-thawed hyperimmune plasma) also exist and have subjectively improved pregnancy rates in repeat breeders. Platelet-rich plasma is a related substance, and recent studies showed IU infusion of platelet-rich plasma caused down-regulation of inflammatory cytokines and improved pregnancy rates in susceptible mares.[44,45] The effects of autologous conditioned serum and mesenchymal allogenic stem cells have also been explored and found to be anti-inflammatory in nature in reproductively normal mares.[46] Mares treated with autologous conditioned serum 24 hours before a dead-sperm challenge had significantly lower neutrophil counts 6 and 24 hours after the challenge. Those treated with mesenchymal allogenic stem cells had significantly lower neutrophil counts 6 hours after sperm challenge relative to control animals. In an earlier study, honing and transplantation of adipose-derived stem cells into the endometrium was demonstrated following IU infusion, but the regenerative effects were not fully explored.[47] It thus seems that the use of generative therapies in equine reproduction is still in a relative nascent stage. More research and clinical studies are necessary to explore further the efficacy and indications for these treatments. Furthermore, and given the current costs, resources, and foresight required to implement these therapies, they are currently deemed novel or adjunctive therapies in cases where conventional treatments have repeatedly failed.

Acupuncture

With its origins in Eastern medicine, acupuncture has been advocated as an adjunctive therapy for various conditions affecting the mare's reproductive tract, including promoting uterine clearance. It is thought to induce uterine contractions and improve tone to help with expulsion of intraluminal fluid. A retrospective study involving 44 broodmares showed a reduction in postmating fluid and improved pregnancy rates in mares with a history of susceptibility.[48] Controlled studies are necessary to compare this modality with more traditional treatments, such as ecbolics and cervical stimulation. Moreover, current acupuncture protocols and methods used (eg, "wet vs dry" needling, electrostimulation) are subject to individual practitioner preferences. Consequently, measuring response is confounded by a lack of control subjects.

Exercise

Although dependent on farm management and limited by space and time, exercise may have many benefits. These include toning of the hindquarters to improve perineal conformation and improved uterine clearance associated with locomotion. In addition, exercise and socialization engage horses mentally and physically. In humans, physical fitness has proven health benefits in staving off the ill effects of advancing age, which is the most significant factor affecting reproductive efficiency in broodmares.[49]

Nutrition

Supplementation with omega-3 fatty acids has become popular and has a small body of research supporting its use. For example, mares fed a commercially available supplement containing docosahexaenoic acid/omega-3 fatty acid (Releira, Arenus, Fort Collins, CO) was associated with a reduction in endometrial cytokine expression in mares bred with frozen semen.[50] Although in need of further study, feeding omega-3 fatty acids has also been postulated to improve follicular and luteal health, which may translate into improved pregnancy and live-foal rates. Certainly no silver-bullet, but use of these omega-3 fatty acids may give an extra edge that can improve the odds of obtaining viable pregnancies.

Antioxidant therapy may be beneficial in staving off sperm membrane damage from free radicals in the seminal plasma or uterus. Hormone-mimicking agents are purported to enhance fertility and/or exert a calming effect. Peer-reviewed studies supporting the use of many of these products are lacking, so further research is necessary to determine the precise value of these products. Furthermore, caution should be exercised in using or mixing supplements because of potential adverse interactions.

REFERENCES

1. USA. What is a *medical* device? FDA basics. Silver Spring (MD): U.S. Food and Drug Administration; 2014.
2. LeBlanc MM, Causey RC. Clinical and subclinical endometritis in the mare: both threats to fertility. Reprod Domest Anim 2009;44:10–22.
3. Troedsson MH. Breeding-induced endometritis in mares. Vet Clin North Am Equine Pract 2006;22:705–12.
4. Ferris RA, McCue PM, Borlee GI, et al. In vitro efficacy of nonantibiotic treatments on biofilm disruption of gram-negative pathogens an in vivo model of infectious endometritis utilizing isolates from the equine uterus. J Clin Microbiol 2016;54:631–9.
5. Gores-Lindholm AR, LeBlanc MM, Causey R, et al. Relationships between intra-uterine infusion of N-acetylcysteine, equine endometrial pathology, neutrophil function, post-breeding therapy, and reproductive performance. Theriogenology 2013;80:218–27.
6. Lyle SK, LeBlanc MM, Staempfli SA, et al. How to use a buffered chelator solution for mares with chronic endometritis. Proceedings of the Annual Convention of the American Association of Equine Practitioners 2011;57:16–8.
7. Stout TAE. Fungal endometritis in the mare. Pferdeheilkunde 2008;1:83–7.
8. Båverud V, Gustafsson A, Franklin A. *Clostridium difficile* associated with acute colitis in mature horses with antibiotics. Equine Vet J 1997;29:279–84.
9. Chambers HF, Bartlett JG, Bonomo RA, et al. Antibacterial resistance leadership group: open for business. Clin Infect Dis 2014;58:1571–6.
10. Pycock JF, Newcombe JR. Assessment of the effect of three treatments to remove intrauterine fluid on pregnancy rate in the mare. Vet Rec 1996;138:320–3.
11. Dascanio JJ. How and when to treat endometritis with systemic or local antibiotics. Proc Ann Conv Amer Assoc Eq Pract 2011;57:24–31.
12. Van Camp SD, Papich MG, Whitacre MD. Administration of ticarcillin in combination with clavulonic acid intravenously and intrauterinely to clinically normal oestrous mares. J Vet Pharmacol Ther 2000;23:373–8.
13. Bermudez V, Sifontes S, Navarro N, et al. Effects of intrauterine infusion of sodium ceftiofur on the endometrium of mares. Proceedings of the Annual Convention of the American Association of Equine Practitioners 1995;41:261–3.
14. Schnobrich MR, Lisa KP, Barber BK, et al. Effects of intrauterine infusion of a water-based suspension of enrofloxacin on mare endometrium. J Equine Vet Sci 2015;35:662–7.

15. Cooke CD. Prophylactic intra-uterine antibacterial therapy. Equine Vet Educ 2015;27:554–5.
16. LeBlanc M, Neuwirth L, Mauragis D, et al. Oxytocin enhances clearance of radio-colloid from the uterine lumen of reproductive normal mares and mares susceptible to endometritis. Equine Vet J 1994;26:279–82.
17. Campbell MLH, England GCW. A comparison of the ecbolic efficacy of intravenous and intrauterine oxytocin treatments. Theriogenology 2002;58:473–7.
18. Sharp DC, Thatcher MJ, Salute ME, et al. Relationship between endometrial oxytocin receptors and oxytocin-induced prostaglandin F2alpha release during the oestrous cycle and early pregnancy in pony mares. J Reprod Fertil 1997;109:137–44.
19. Paccamonti DL, Pycock JF, Taverne MAM, et al. PGFM response to exogenous oxytocin and determination of the half-life of oxytocin in nonpregnant mares. Equine Vet J 1999;31:285–8.
20. Schramme AR, Pinto CR, Davis J, et al. Pharmacokinetics of carbetocin, a long-acting oxytocin analogue, following intravenous administration in horses. Equine Vet J 2008;40:658–61.
21. Combs GB, LeBlanc MM, Neuwirth L, et al. Effects of prostaglandin F2alpha, cloprostenol and fenprostalene on uterine clearance of radiocolloid in the mare. Theriogenology 1996;45:1449–55.
22. Nie GJ, Johnson KE, Wenzel JGW, et al. Effect of periovulatory ecbolics on luteal function and fertility. Theriogenology 2002;58:461–3.
23. von Reitzenstein M, Callahan MA, Hansen PJ, et al. Aberrations in uterine contractile patterns in mares with delayed uterine clearance after administration of detomidine and oxytocin. Theriogenology 2002;58:887–98.
24. Cuervo-Arango J, Domingo-Ortiz R. Systemic treatment with high dose of flunixin meglumine is able to block ovulation by inducing hemorrhage and luteinisation of follicles. Theriogenology 2011;75:707–14.
25. Livini M, Zamboni A, Necchi D. Effect of pre-insemination uterine lavage on fertility in a population of subfertile mares. Annual Conference of the American Association of Equine Practitioners 2013;59:514–6.
26. Vanderwall DK, Woods GL. Effect on fertility of uterine lavage performed immediately prior to insemination in mares. J Am Vet Med Assoc 2003;222:1108–10.
27. Brinsko SP, Varner DD, Blanchard TL. The effect of uterine lavage performed four hours post insemination on pregnancy rate in mares. Theriogenology 1992;35:1111–9.
28. Bucca S, Carli A, Buckley T, et al. The use of dexamethasone administered to mares at breeding time in the modulation of persistent mating induced endometritis. Theriogenology 2008;70:1093–100.
29. Dell'Aqua JA Jr, Papa FO, Lopes MD, et al. Modulation of acute uterine inflammatory response after artificial insemination with equine frozen semen. Anim Reprod Sci 2006;94:270–3.
30. Rogan D, Fumuso E, Rodriguez E, et al. Use of a mycobacterial cell wall extract (MCWE) in susceptible mares to clear experimentally induced endometritis with *Streptococcus zooepidemicus*. J Equine Vet Sci 2007;27:112–7.
31. Rohrbach BW, Sheerin PC, Cantrell CK, et al. Effect of adjunctive treatment with intravenously administered *Proprionibacterium acnes* on reproductive performance in mares with persistent endometritis. J Am Vet Med Assoc 2007;231:107–13.
32. Petersen MR, Lu K, Christoffersen M, et al. Impact of activation and subsequent antimicrobial treatment of dormant endometrial streptococci in the Thoroughbred problem mare: a descriptive study. Proceedings of the Annual Convention of the Society for Theriogenology 2013;5:408.

33. Petersen MR, Skive B, Christoffersen M, et al. Activation of persistent *Strepto-coccus equi* subspecies *zooepidemicus* in mares with subclinical endometritis. Vet Microbiol 2015;179:119–25.

34. Petersen MR, Nielsen JM, Lehn-Jensen H, et al. *Streptococcus equi* subspecies zooepidemicus resides deep in the chronically infected endometrium of mares. Clinical Theriogenology 2009;1:393–409.

35. LeBlanc MM, McKinnon AO. Breeding the problem mare. In: McKinnon AO, Squires EL, Vaala WE, et al, editors. Equine reproduction. Ames (IA): Wiley-Black-well; 2011. p. 2620–42.

36. Ferris R. Bacterial endometritis: a focus on biofilms. Clinical Theriogenology 2014;6:315–9.

37. Hassett DJ, Ma JF, Elkins JG, et al. Quorum sensing in *Pseudomonas aeruginosa* controls expression of catalase and superoxide dismutase genes and mediates biofilm susceptibility to hydrogen peroxide. Mol Microbiol 1999;34:1082–93.

38. Witte TS, Melkus E, Walter I, et al. Effects of oral treatment with *N*-acetylcysteine on the viscosity of intrauterine mucus and endometrial function in estrous mares. Theriogenology 2012;78:1199–208.

39. LeBlanc M. Advances in the diagnosis and treatment of chronic infectious and post-mating-induced endometritis in the mare. Reprod Domest Anim 2010;45: 21–7.

40. Weinstein WL, Moore PA, Sanchez S, et al. In vitro efficacy of a buffered chelating solution as an antimicrobial potentiator for antifungal drugs against fungal pathogens obtained from horses with mycotic keratitis. Am J Vet Res 2006;67:562–8.

41. Bracher V, Neuschaefer A, Allen WR. The effect of intra-uterine infusion of kero-sene on the endometrium of mares. J Reprod Fertil Suppl 1991;44:706–7.

42. Bradecamp EA, Ahlschwede SA, Cook JL. The effects of intra-uterine kero-sene infusion on endometrial epithelial cilia concentration. J Equine Vet Sci 2014;34:134.

43. Pascoe DR. Effect of adding autologous plasma to an intrauterine antibiotic ther-apy after breeding on pregnancy rates in mares. Biol Reprod 1995;Monograph Series 1:539–43.

44. Metcalf ES, Scoggin K, Troedsson MHT. The effect of platelet-rich plasma on endometrial pro-inflammatory cytokines in susceptible mares following semen deposition. J Equine Vet Sci 2012;32:475–518.

45. Metcalf ES. The effect of platelet-rich plasma (PRP) on intraluminal fluid and preg-nancy rates in mares susceptible to persistent mating-induced endometritis. J Equine Vet Sci 2014;34:128.

46. Ferris RA, Frisbie DD, McCue PM. Use of mesenchymal stem cells or autologous conditioned serum to modulate the inflammatory response to spermatozoa in ma-res. Theriogenology 2014;82:36–42.

47. Mambelli LI, Winter GH, Kerkis A, et al. A novel strategy of mesenchymal stem cells delivery in the uterus of mares with endometriosis. Theriogenology 2013; 79:744–50.

48. Rathgeber R. Acupuncture therapies for equine reproductive disorders. Hagyard Bluegrass Symposium. Lexington, October 25–28, 2000.

49. Scoggin C. Not just a number: effect of age on fertility, pregnancy and offspring vigour in thoroughbred brood-mares. Reprod Fertil Dev 2015;27:872–9.

50. Brendemuehl JP, Kopp K, Altman J. Influence of dietary algal N-3 fatty acids on breeding induced inflammation and endometrial cytokine expression in mares bred with frozen semen. J Equine Vet Sci 2014;34:123–4.

Advances in Diagnostics and Therapeutic Techniques in Breeding Behavior Disorders in Stallions

Sue M. McDonnell, MA, PhD

KEYWORDS

• Stallion • Sexual behavior • Breeding disorders

INTRODUCTION

Despite the suboptimal aspects of domestic breeding conditions compared to the natural conditions under which their reproductive behavior evolved, most domestic stallions have little difficulty adapting to any number of various management and breeding programs. Most immediately respond adequately or quickly learn to safely abide the restraint and direction imposed by a human handler, and can usually adapt to changes of methods of breeding for semen collection, housing, handling, social, and other management conditions. For those that do not, the problems can range from inadequate or variable sexual interest and response to overenthusiastic or aggressive response beyond the ability of the handlers to safely direct and control.

INADEQUATE SEXUAL INTEREST AND AROUSAL
Slow-Starting Novice Breeders

One of the more common problems for stallions during first introduction to breeding is inadequate sexual interest or response. Some may seem interested but are slow to achieve and/or maintain an erection. Some seem confused or conflicted, and easily distracted by ordinary environmental sounds or activities or reactions of the mare. Some may initially seem interested but quickly lose interest. Some may achieve erection but then not proceed normally to mount, or may mount and seem confused about how to proceed.

Inherent temperament in regard to breeding style and stamina naturally varies among individuals, and this factor may account for the difficulties of some slow-starting novice breeders. In the case of inadequate sexual behavior, the more

No conflicts of interest.

Department of Clinical Studies, New Bolton Center, Section of Reproduction and Behavior, University of Pennsylvania School of Veterinary Medicine, 382 West Street Road, Kennett Square, PA 19348, USA

E-mail address: suemcd@vet.upenn.edu

Vet Clin Equine 32 (2016) 513–519
http://dx.doi.org/10.1016/j.cveq.2016.07.008
0749-0739/16/© 2016 Elsevier Inc. All rights reserved.

important factors likely contributing to inadequate response in the domestic environment are the numerous management, training, and breeding practices that tend to adversely affect normal expression of sexual behavior of stallions. For example, through the training and performance years, colts and young stallions are typically actively discouraged from expressing sexual interest and response. Although most stallions can quickly learn to distinguish breeding opportunities from performance or training, this experienced-based suppression of sexual behavior likely plays a considerable role in the inadequate response of many novice breeders. Similarly, many stallions are punished for exhibiting normal spontaneous erection and penile movements, often called masturbation. It has been shown that punishment of this normal frequent behavior adversely affects breeding behavior.[1] In addition, in natural herds, the behavior, endocrinology, and fertility of individual stallions is naturally affected by their bachelor or harem social status within the herd at any time.[2,3] Certain stallions hold harem status with access to breeding of their harem mares, whereas other stallions, known as bachelor stallions, do not hold regular access to mares. Some bachelors gain access to breeding via the alternate breeding strategy and style known as sneak breeding. Modulation of reproductive function of stallions can occur under domestic conditions and so is another important factor in instances of inadequate sexual interest and response in domestic breeding environments.

Another consideration is the style and expertise of the handling for breeding to which the stallion is exposed. Stallion behavior can be considerably influenced, positively or negatively, by the skill and style of mare and stallion handling for breeding. In addition, certain aspects of the physical facility where breeding is done can seem to affect mare and stallion behavior positively or negatively.

Regardless of these and other potential factors, most slow-starting stallions respond well with simple management and handling changes, as opposed to more complicated behavior modification regimens or pharmacologic therapies. The general approach is to try to identify and address any contributing factors. The following is a list of recommended considerations for assisting a slow-starting novice breeder:

1. Evaluate and address any potential discomfort or health problems that may be contributing to a stallion's insecurity in the breeding situation.
2. House and breed away from any other stallions.
3. Provide generous exposure to mares, as continuously and directly as safely possible.
4. For breeding stimulus or mount mares, provide those that seem to be most stimulating to the particular stallion. Almost all stallions show greater interest and respond more vigorously to intact mares compared with ovariectomized mares, regardless of their receptivity. The response is also usually greater for mares that are cycling naturally, as opposed to those that have been exposed to cycle manipulation or ovulation-induction agents. For many stallions, response tends to be greater with mares closer to ovulation as opposed to early estrus. Avoid washing the perineum or wrapping the tail. These may alter the natural visual and olfactory stimuli. Avoid odors of other stallions that may be intimidating to a low-confidence stallion, for example, from test mounting. Minimal restraint will allow the mare to show the natural estrus postures and movements that are generally most stimulating to stallions. **Fig. 1** illustrates the change from normal estrus to more aggressive type posture resulting from restraint. Breeding boots and hobbles can cause the mare to step in an unnatural gait that can startle stallions. **Fig. 2** illustrates the head-turned- back posture representing the natural mating invitation gesture of mares. Allowing and encouraging a stimulus mare to express this posture can immediate stimulate otherwise reluctant stallions.

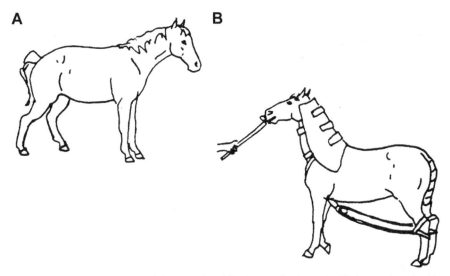

Fig. 1. Normal estrus posture (A) versus head high, ears back, and tail clamped evoked by twitch (B).

5. Assess and consider improvements to the breeding environment. Example aspects to consider include minimal potentially distracting activities, quiet nonslip footing, ample ceiling height, and no reflective glass in which the stallion may perceive his own reflection as another intimidating stallion. Outdoor breeding areas away from the sight or sound of other stallions often eliminate many of the features of indoor breeding rooms that seem to be worrisome to slow-starting novices. If using a dummy mount, evaluate for and address any features that can be improved to reduce inhibition of the stallion.[4]

6. Assess and consider improvements in animal handling, both mare and stallion. Aspects that typically improve the stallion's sexual response include minimum effective restraint on the stallion and mare, minimum personnel, calm and organized manner, minimum punitive reaction to any awkward moves or perceived

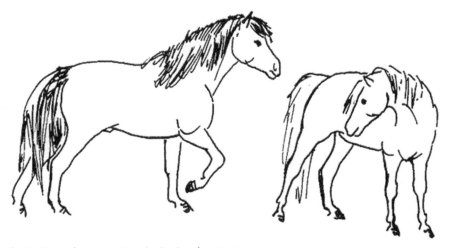

Fig. 2. Natural mare mating invitational posture.

misbehavior, careful respectful nonconfrontational guidance of the stallion with a well-fitted stout stallion halter so as to minimize adverse consequences to either the stallion or mare from normal natural elements of the precopulatory sequence (eg, striking, nipping), mounting without erection, awkward mounting, or normal frustration responses (eg, head tossing, spinning, and kick threat toward mare, displaced aggression toward handler).

7. Evaluate and abide any apparent preferences and aversions until the stallion gets some successful experience to build his confidence. Mare preferences can include such aspects as particular breed, color, maiden or foaling mare, or stage of estrus.

8. Treatment with anxiolytics can be helpful to release inhibition of sexual behavior. Diazepam (0.05 mg/kg, administered as a slow intravenous injection about 5–7 minutes before expected mounting) is helpful in many instances.[5] Anxiolytic therapy may also release aggressive behavior from inhibition, such that stallions may be characteristically quick to show colt-like aggression, as if they have forgotten their ground manners. This can complicate handling. Discipline for this aggression when trying to build a stallion's sexual confidence can be counterproductive.

9. Whether or not testosterone levels are within the range of normal, increasing circulating levels usually increases sexual motivation and response. Increasing androgen naturally by providing exposure to mares and freedom from exposure to other stallions is typically quite effective and preferable, with little worry of adverse effects on endogenous facility. Alternatively, circulating androgens can be increased by administering gonadotropin-releasing hormone (GnRH), human chorionic gonadotropin (hCG), or testosterone. Of these methods, GnRH (50 μg simple decapeptide administered subcutaneously 2 hours and again 1 hour before each breeding session) usually results in concentrations that are double the baseline at the time of the session. Administration of a single dose of hCG (10,000 IU intravenously) results in increased circulating testosterone for up to a week or longer, often with the peak levels at 3 days after administration (McDonnell, unpublished, 2009). Testosterone supplementation can be administered intramuscularly, subcutaneously, or trandermally. Depending on the formulation and route of delivery, circulating levels can vary widely among individual stallions with any given regimen. It is advisable to carefully monitor with frequent assays to avoid reaching high levels (>4 ng/mL). Of these 3 methods of increasing circulating testosterone, the GnRH regimen before each session is believed to be the least likely to adversely affect endogenous endocrinology and fertility. Increasing testosterone by any of these methods often also promotes undesirable aggressive tendencies that can complicate handling and mare receptivity.

Experienced Breeders

Inadequate breeding behavior in an otherwise normal experienced breeder can take the form of gradually diminishing interest, slowing or variable response, or can be an abrupt loss of interest and response. The problem can be seasonal, in that the stallion is especially slow in the winter months of the early breeding season. For stallions with a heavy breeding schedule, problems may be associated with the later or heaviest workload portion of the breeding season.

Diminished sexual arousal and response may result from changes in management and handling factors similar to those affect novice breeders. For stallions with a change in interest and arousal after having no behavior problems for years, physical discomfort and other health-related factors are often at play.

Recommendations listed for the slow-starting novice can be considered for helping the experienced stallion that develops behavior problems.

OVERENTHUSIASTIC, DIFFICULT-TO-CONTROL BREEDING BEHAVIOR

Urgency to breed and style of interaction with a mare and handler vary widely among domestic stallions. Normal breeding behavior of stallions living under natural herd social conditions or in long-term pasture breeding arrangements is much less variable. The behavior of most stallions breeding at liberty is relatively quiet, relaxed, and methodical compared with that of many domestic stallions when bred in-hand. Rearing, charging toward a mare, or serious biting and striking, are not normal under free-breeding conditions. The high urgency and boisterous response of many hand-bred stallions is likely attributable to unnatural separation from mares, with only momentary access before breeding, along with limited precopulatory interaction inherent to in-hand direction and physical restraint of the mare, as well as the stallion, during the breeding itself. Aggressive behaviors toward the handler or the mare are also almost always the result of human handling. Much of the variation in style of breeding among stallions more or less reflects the level of skill of the handling team and the breeding atmosphere to which the stallion is exposed.

Most stallions, no matter how urgent, can improve with schooling by a skilled handling team. For stallions whose behavior and breeding style are beyond the skills of the handling team or particular facilities, schooling of the stallion and the handlers by a professional stallion-handling team skilled in nonconfrontational stallion handling is advised.

For most overenthusiastic stallions, a period of intense schooling can result in considerable improvement. Intensive repetition of the breeding routine, with ejaculation as many as several times per day for several consecutive days will lower the urgency to the point at which the stallion is better able to understand the routine and learn to trust that the handler will get him to the goal. Specific refinement goals, such as organized approach to the mare at the pace of the handler, tolerating manipulation of the genitals and other procedure delays, and organized mount and dismount, can be the aim of each successive session. After a period of sexual rest, stallions will again be somewhat fresh and highly aroused but often seem less urgent or aggressive, as well as more willing to cooperate with human handling and the controlled breeding routine.

By trial and error, sometimes alternate housing arrangements can be found to reduce the urgency to breed and tendencies for aggression in the breeding situation. Housing near mares will generally increase testosterone, increasing arousal and aggression. Housing near more dominant stallions and away from mares generally reduces testosterone and subdues arousal.

Severe restraint or punitive methods of behavior modification are often counterproductive, and so generally not advised. Harsh restraint, such as war bridles or heavily confining breeding bridles, can further provoke explosive aggression to dangerous or savage levels. Alternatively, harsh restraint and discipline can create severely inadequate sexual interest and response. In general a well-designed, well-fitted stallion breeding halter as shown in **Fig. 3**, with a soft brass chain lead through the mouth or over the noseband, is sufficient for guiding a highly motivated, aroused stallion. When necessary, in skilled hands, a humanely applied gum chain of soft brass or covered with plastic tubing, can sufficiently quiet and respectfully guide most superurgent stallions.

When schooling a stallion, it can be helpful to reduce the stimulation of the breeding situation when possible. For example, for semen collection, a stimulus mare can be eliminated. If needed, estrous mare urine can be substituted to elicit arousal, or a mare can be presented at a distance or partially behind a barrier. For schooling for natural cover, an ovariectomized mare is usually less stimulating than a naturally cycling mare. For stallions to be bred by natural cover, use of a dummy mount and artificial vagina can be useful during schooling phase. Once the stallion has become

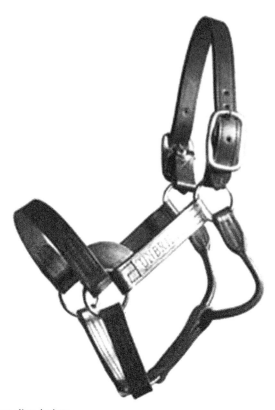

Fig. 3. Stallion breeding halter.

organized, the stimulation can be gradually increased while reinforcing patience with the routine.

In extremely challenging cases, impairing vision with blinker or full cup blinders, as shown in **Fig. 4**, can sometimes sufficiently reduce stimulation, yet allow safe handling. Visually impaired stallions may require expert handling skills. Certainly before using visual impairment in the breeding context, the stallion should be

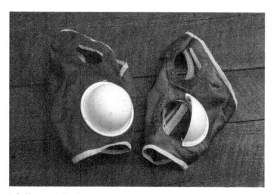

Fig. 4. Blinkers and full cup blinders.

acclimated in a nonsexual setting to assess the stallion's behavior and the handler's ability to safely direct the visually impaired stallion.

REFERENCES

1. McDonnell SM, Hinze AL. Aversive conditioning of periodic spontaneous erection adversely affects sexual behavior and semen in stallions. Anim Reprod Sci 2005; 89:77–92.
2. McDonnell SM, Murray SC. Bachelor and harem stallion behavior and endocrinology. Biol Reprod Monogr 1995;1:135–48.
3. McDonnell SM. The equid ethogram: practical field guide to horse behavior. Lexington (KY): Blood Horse Publications; 2003.
4. McDonnell SM. How to select and fit a breeding dummy mount for stallions. AAEP Proceedings 2001;47:417–9.
5. McDonnell SM, Kenney RM, Meckley PE, et al. Conditioned suppression of sexual behavior in stallions and reversal with diazepam. Phyiol Behav 1985;34(6):951–6.

Advances in Stallion Semen Cryopreservation

Marco Antonio Alvarenga, DVM, PhD*, Frederico Ozanam Papa, DVM, PhD,
Carlos Ramires Neto, DVM, MS

KEYWORDS

- Stallion • Frozen semen • Sperm selection • Epididymal sperm • Centrifugation
- Cushion • Spermfilter

KEY POINTS

- Recent advances in extender composition have allowed increased quality and fertility of frozen stallion semen from ejaculated and epidydimal sperm.
- The use of new laboratory techniques to select and better protect sperm cells has allowed successful freezing of semen from stallions with sperm more susceptible to damage during the freezing-thawing process.
- Different quality control tests are available to better determine the quality of frozen semen. However, there is no reliable in vitro test to predict fertility.

INTRODUCTION

The use of stallion frozen semen minimizes the spread of disease, eliminates geographic barriers, and preserves the genetic material of the animal for unlimited time. Significant progress in the process of frozen thawed stallion semen and consequently fertility has been achieved over the last decade. Progress has been associated with the use of (1) new AI techniques, such as deep uterine artificial insemination (AI), which permits the use of a small number of sperm cells; (2) other cryoprotectants than glycerol and new commercially available extenders that results in better sperm cryo-survival; and (3) sperm selection techniques to increase the quality of frozen semen. New laboratory approaches are also available to evaluate and overcome the deleterious effects of cryopreservation.

These improvements not only increased fertility rates but also allowed cryopreservation of semen from "poor freezer" stallions, inducing a positive impact in the interest of different horse breed associations and owners in the use of stallion frozen semen

Department of Animal Reproduction and Veterinary Radiology, São Paulo State University—UNESP, Botucatu, Brazil
* Corresponding author. Department of Animal Reproduction and Veterinary Radiology, São Paulo State University-UNESP, PO BOX 560, Botucatu, São Paulo 18618970, Brazil.
E-mail address: malvarenga.fmvz.unesp.br@gmail.com

Vet Clin Equine 32 (2016) 521–530
http://dx.doi.org/10.1016/j.cveq.2016.08.003
0749-0739/16/© 2016 Elsevier Inc. All rights reserved.

vetequine.theclinics.com

with thousands of mares being inseminated yearly worldwide. Approximately 20% of embryo donor mares have been bred in Brazil with frozen semen and 90% of foals from Standardbred mares are produced by AI in Australia[1] with frozen or cooled semen.

This article reviews traditional steps and new strategies for stallion semen handling and processing, which are performed to overcome the deleterious effects of semen preservation and consequently improve frozen semen quality and fertility.

PROCESSING SEMEN FOR FREEZING

After collection, semen must be filtered to remove the gelatinous portion and debris from the ejaculate. Semen must then be diluted with skim milk base extender and evaluated for motility, viability, and sperm concentration to determine the number of straws. After this, centrifugation is performed to remove the seminal plasma and the sperm pellet is resuspended in extender containing cryoprotectant to the volume required to achieve the desired concentration. Finally, semen is loaded into straws. It is recommended after this time to perform a new analysis of motility, viability, and sperm concentration to ensure the quality and quantity of sperm placed in each straw. Next, semen is frozen using a predetermined freezing curve according to the medium to be used. The straws are stored in liquid nitrogen containers until thawing and used for insemination. It is recommended to perform another analysis of motility and sperm viability after thawing, to verify the quality of the semen to be inseminated (**Fig. 1**).

Standard Procedures for Semen Collection

The penis should be washed, especially the urethral fossa, with warm water to eliminate smegma and microorganisms just before collection. It is important to avoid the use of bactericidal solutions that can disrupt the normal bacterial flora from the penis.

The two most traditional methods to collect semen from a stallion involve the use of a phantom or a mare in heat. The use of phantoms is safest for the animal and operator and stallions can easily be trained to perform a collection into an artificial vagina.

There are different models of artificial vagina available to collect semen from stallions. The Missouri and Colorado models in the United States, Hannover in Europe,

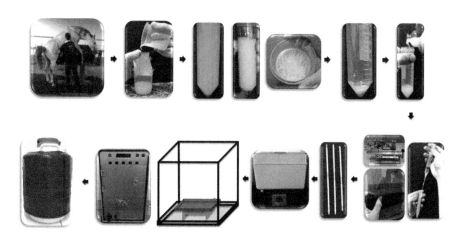

Fig. 1. Steps in the semen freezing process. First the semen is collected, filtered to remove gel, and diluted with milk-skimmed media extender. After seminal plasma is removed, the pellet of sperm is resuspended with freezing extender and finally frozen.

and Botucatu in Brazil are the most widely used models. These models are all based on the concept of a bladder filled with hot/warm water to provide adequate pressure and temperature to stimulate stallions to ejaculate. The use of a disposable plastic inner liner is strongly recommended for sanitary reasons. Stallions can harbor potential pathogens on the penis, such as *Pseudomonas*, which can be transmitted to the mare during breeding. Caution should also be taken with the use of latex artificial vagina (AV) inner liners because they may be toxic when in contact with the sperm, especially when these liners are new.

The artificial vagina must be filled with hot water at around 50°C and may or may not be lubricated using a neutral lubricant gel. We have chosen not to use lubricants in our laboratory because many lubricants can induce damage to the sperm.

Another method to perform semen collection is with the animal on the ground. This technique is recommended for stallions with musculoskeletal problems that are unable to do a safe mount. This technique exposes the operator to greater risk and therefore must be performed with caution. The animal should be stimulated by a mare in heat properly contained and the artificial vagina should be introduced over the penis, allowing the stallion perform pelvic thrusts and ejaculate.

Dilution of Semen After Collection

The gel-free semen must be diluted with a skim milk– or casein-based extender. This dilution should be at minimum of 1:1 ration (vol/vol). When working with very concentrated semen, it is recommended to perform greater dilutions (2:1) to reduce damage and sperm loss during removal of seminal plasma. The diluent medium should be added to the semen and must be preheated to 37°C to avoid cold shock.

There is a wide variety of commercial skimmed milk– or casein-based extenders for horse semen. They provide the necessary nutrients for sperm metabolism, function as buffers to maintain the proper pH and osmolality control, and also protect the plasma membrane against cold shock and oxidative damage. Furthermore, because of the presence of antibiotics, these extenders play an important role in preventing bacterial growth.

How to Concentrate the Sperm

The seminal plasma is mostly produced by the accessory sex glands and expelled in fractions during ejaculation. This carries fluid and sperm, and also participates in the sperm capacitation process.[2] The high volume of stallion ejaculate makes it necessary to remove them before cryopreservation.

Centrifugation is the most common technique used for concentrating sperm from a stallion ejaculate. Some studies, however, point to the damaging effects of centrifugation on the sperm: the force and duration of centrifugation required to remove the seminal plasma might negatively affect sperm motility, integrity, and recovery rate.

To remove the seminal plasma via conventional centrifugation, semen diluted with extender is placed in 50-mL conical tubes and loaded in a centrifuge. The force and time of centrifugation may negatively impact on motility, integrity, and sperm recovery rate. High centrifugal forces cause strong adhesion of the pellet, which is harmful to sperm cell, whereas low forces promote low recovery of sperm. In our experience the best combination of force and time for a good sperm recovery rate and less damage to sperm quality is $600 \times g$ for 10 minutes.[3]

Immediately after centrifugation, the supernatant must be removed using a disposable catheter or needle coupled with a syringe or vacuum pump, and the pellet resuspended in the selected cryopreservation extender. If the resulting pellet is too compacted, the centrifugation force should be reduced in subsequent collections, or other techniques should be used to minimize excessive sperm packing.

An alternative method for removing seminal plasma from ejaculate aiming to minimizing sperm damage is the cushioned centrifugation technique. This method attempts to maximize sperm recovery from centrifuged equine semen by using high centrifugation forces, and preventing damage with a cushion fluid placed at the bottom of the centrifuge tube.[4]

Three commercial products are available: Eqcellsire (IMV, Lisieux, France), Cushion Fluid (Minitube, Tiefenbach,Germany), and more recently Red Cushion (Botupharma, Botucatu, Brazil). Red Cushion is a red solution that allows better visualization of the concentrated sperm pellet.

To remove the seminal plasma using cushioned centrifugation, semen must be diluted 1:1 with a skim milk–based extender and placed in a 50-mL conical tube. One to five mL of cushion is carefully placed in the bottom of the tube using a catheter coupled with a syringe, and centrifugation is performed at $1000 \times g$ for 20 minutes.[5]

Following centrifugation, the supernatant must be carefully removed via aspiration using a catheter coupled with a syringe or a vacuum pump. Next, the cushion fluid is carefully removed using a catheter, and the pellet resuspended in the desired extender (**Fig. 2**).

An alternative to the use of centrifugation to concentrate sperm is to filter the semen through a synthetic hydrophilic membrane (Sperm Filter, Botupharma, Botucatu, Brazil), which retains sperm and allows only the removal of seminal plasma.[6] Raw semen must be diluted two parts semen and one part skim milk–based extender, placed on the filter, and using gentle motion the filter is touched against the surface of a 25-cm Petri dish. The pore size and capillarity of the filter are such that the seminal plasma flows through, but the sperm are retained on the membrane. A predetermined volume of freezing extender is then added to the filter, and the mixture is homogenized to resuspend the sperm. The entire process lasts 5 to 10 minutes, and the same filter may be used up to 10 times for the same stallion without affecting sperm quality and recovery. The filter has also the advantage of not requiring centrifugation, which can cause mechanic damage to sperm cells (**Fig. 3**).

Adding the Freezing Extender

In general the extenders used for freezing semen are composed of substances to stabilize the pH, neutralize the toxic products produced by sperm metabolism, protect

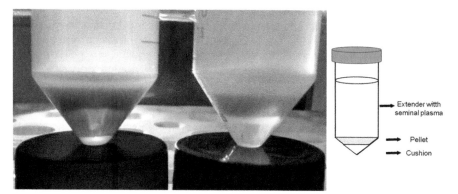

Extender witth seminal plasma

Pellet

Cushion

Fig. 2. Differences between the use of Red Cushion and conventional cushion fluid to centrifugate equine semen.

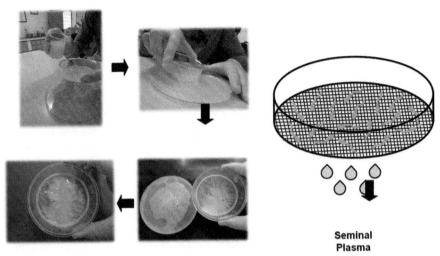

Seminal Plasma

Fig. 3. Steps and schematic design for the use of Sperm Filter to remove seminal plasma.

against thermal shock, maintain the electrolytic and osmotic balance, inhibit bacterial growth, and supply energy. The extenders must also contain cryoprotectants to prevent the formation of intracellular and extracellular ice. Several commercial extenders are available, the most common being Lactose EDTA (Animal Reproduction Systems, Chino, CA), INRA freeze (IMV), and BotuCrio (Botupharma).

Several cryoprotectants have been used to freeze stallion semen. These cryoprotectants are classified as penetrating or nonpenetrating and as intracellular or extracellular. The intracellular cryoprotectants act via their ability to bind water or their colligative properties. The extracellular agents protect the sperm cells using osmotic effects to create a hypertonic environment that induces the movement of water out of the cells, dehydrating the sperm and reducing the chances for ice crystals to form inside the cells. Thus, sperm damage caused by ice formation is prevented. The nonpenetrating cryoprotectants are efficient in protecting the sperm cells during freezing without penetration. Some examples include egg yolk, milk, and some sugars.

Over the past 65 years egg yolk has been routinely used as extenders for the cryopreservation of mammalian semen and to protect sperm against thermal shock, because of the presence of low-density lipoproteins in egg yolk. These lipoproteins adhere to the cell membrane during freezing, restoring the lost phospholipids. The egg yolk seemingly induces a transient change in the composition of the phospholipids to prevent the rupture of the cell membrane and protect the sperm cells. Generally, egg yolk is used at a concentration of 20%.

Sugars provide another type of nonpenetrating cryoprotection; they act on the osmotic pressure dehydrating the cells, and thus reduce the amount of intracellular water available for potential ice formation. In addition, sugars are an energy source for the sperm during incubation and protect the plasma membrane during freezing and thawing by direct interaction with the cell membrane.

Glycerol is the universal cryoprotectant used for the cryopreservation of semen. Glycerol penetrates the cell membrane by passive diffusion and remain in the membrane and cytoplasm. Although these substances cross the cell membrane until equilibrium is reached, the movement of water occurs more rapidly and causes cell dehydration. In addition to its undesirable osmotic effects, glycerol may exert direct action on the cell membrane, where it binds to the phospholipid head groups reducing the membrane fluidity.

Methylformamide has also been used and, in our experience, it causes less osmotic damage to sperm than glycerol because of the lower molecular weight and viscosity.[7] For stallions with semen that has satisfactory freezability ("good freezers"), the use of extenders containing dimethylformamide and methylformamide may not result in a significant increase in postthaw sperm motility; however, it does increase the fertility of the frozen semen. In stallions whose semen has low resistance to cryopreservation ("bad freezers"), the use of extenders containing dimethylformamide and methylformamide provides a significant improvement in sperm motility and fertility compared with extenders containing glycerol.

The use of a combination of cryoprotectants affords better protection to sperm compared with the use of single agents. Several equine reproduction centers in Europe, the United States, and Brazil have preferentially used a commercial extender (BotuCrio), which includes a combination of methylformamide and glycerol.

The extender used in cryopreservation must be added to the semen immediately after removal of the seminal plasma. The total number of sperm in the recovered semen sample must be determined to calculate the final volume of extender required. Usually, stallion sperm are cryopreserved at a concentration between 200 and 400 $\times$ 10^6 sperm/mL or 100 and 200 $\times$ 10^6 sperm per 0.5-mL straw.

Packaging

After removal of seminal plasma and addition of the appropriated extender, the semen must be packed. Currently, semen is packaged in plastic straws with a volume of 0.5 mL or 0.25 mL.

Semen is loaded into straws using automated equipment (costly) or manually. Once filled, the straws must be sealed using one of several techniques available, such as polyvinyl alcohol powder, metal and glass balls, or ultrasonic sealers. Is important to have an air bubble in the center of the straw to allow for expansion of the fluid during cryopreservation and avoid rupture of the straw during thawing.

Freezing Curves

Once the semen is packaged, the process of cooling samples to 5°C begins. The time required to achieve equilibrium at 5°C varies according to the extender used and the manufacturer's instructions. The freezing process must be slow enough to allow cell dehydration, avoiding the formation of intracellular ice crystals, and quick enough to prevent sperm exposure to supersaturated solutions as the extracellular water freezes.

The freezing curve must be performed in two steps: first the semen straws are cooled from room temperature to 5°C at a rate of 3°C to 5°C per minute, and then they are frozen to −196°C at a rate of 20 to 50°C per minute.

There are particularities between extenders in the protocol to freeze stallion semen. For INRA 96, the laboratory recommends cooling for 2 hours at 5°C before starting the freezing process. For BotuCrio, a faster equilibration time is recommended (20 minutes at 5°C). The recommended freezing curve after the equilibration is similar between extenders.

Two techniques are available for freezing equine semen: one uses Styrofoam coolers, and the other uses programmable semen freezer machines. Studies comparing both freezing techniques found no differences between them; however, the use of programmable systems provides better control of all procedures described previously.

We prefer to use a 45-L Styrofoam box filled with liquid nitrogen and the straws are placed in a floating rack at 3 cm above the liquid nitrogen. It is important to have sufficient liquid nitrogen to keep the temperature stable for the duration of the procedure and also allow at least 3 minutes with the lid closed before placing the straws over the liquid nitrogen.

Thawing and Postthaw Semen Analysis

Several protocols are available for thawing equine semen. Some studies indicate that temperatures and times of 46°C for 20 seconds or 37°C for 1 minute are the most appropriate protocols for 0.5-mL straws. Redilution of the semen after thawing must be avoided because it can induce osmotic damage to the cell.

Semen should be evaluated after thawing for determination of sperm motility (total and progressive), sperm morphology, vigor of sperm movement, and the number of sperm cells per straw.

For semen with acceptable postthaw motility but low fertility, we recommend the use of more sophisticated methods for semen analysis, such as analysis of the cell membrane integrity, and DNA analysis via flow cytometry.[8] Acceptable parameters for postthaw semen quality are more than 50% of total motility, more than 30% of progressive motility, and expected fertility rates of 40% to 60% per cycle.

Insemination Using Frozen Semen

The ideal window of time for insemination using frozen semen is from 12 hours before to 6 hours after ovulation. Management of mares for insemination with frozen semen requires daily ultrasonographic evaluation during estrus and the induction of ovulation using human chorionic gonadotropin (1500 IU) or gonadotropin-releasing hormone (deslorelin acetate, 1 mg) once a follicle larger than 35 mm is detected in the presence of uterine edema. Twenty-four hours after inducing ovulation, ultrasound evaluation must be performed every 6 hours and insemination is performed once ovulation is detected. Alternatively, insemination is performed at fixed times at 24 and 40 hours or at 30 and 48 after induction of ovulation. In our AI protocol we routinely induce ovulation between 9 and 10 PM and expect ovulation during the day (between 32 and 48 hours after hormonal treatment), avoiding inseminations in the middle of the night.

STRATEGIES TO IMPROVE SEMEN QUALITY

Selection of stallion is performed by phenotypic assessments, such as the conformation of the animal and their athletic performance,[9] unlike bovines where reproductive parameters are assessed in bulls before becoming a commercial sire. Another factor that affects sperm quality is age, and often owners decide to freeze semen from stallions that have advanced age and may be subfertile.

Several techniques have been developed to increase the sperm quality of stallions. Stallions whose semen does not resist the centrifugation process, the use of such techniques as SpermFilter, and cushioned centrifugation may be beneficial. For stallions whose semen has a low resistance to cryopreservation, the use of extenders with specific cryoprotectants, such as amines, may improve sperm cryosurvival.

When the initial quality of semen is poor, sperm selection using commercially available density gradients, such as EquiPure (Nidacon, Gothenburg, Sweden) or Androcoll-E (Minitube) can be performed before cryopreservation.[10,11] These gradients select the sperm that exhibit progressive motility, cell integrity, and no morphologic defects (**Fig. 4**).

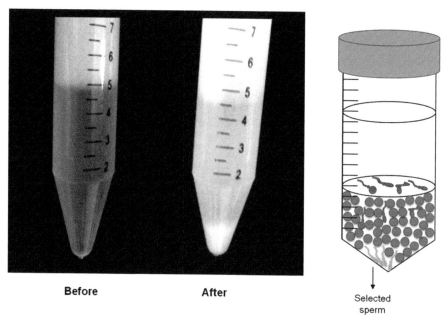

Before   After   Selected sperm

Fig. 4. Image of the semen before and after centrifugation with Equipure.

Another alternative is to select sperm after thawing. For this procedure, the contents of four straws are gently layered on top of 2 mL of Equipure, centrifuged at 300 g for 20 minutes, and the pellet resuspended with the freezing extender. Based in our experience this protocol improves the motility and the fertility of some stallions (unpublished data). It is postulated that the removal of bad quality or dead sperm that can generate oxidative reagents can improve the fertility.

FREEZING OF EPIDIDYMAL SEMEN

Epididymal sperm cryopreservation is the last chance to preserve the semen from a stallion. Following death or castration, the sperm can remain viable in the epididymis for 24 to 48 hours. In stallions exhibiting severe toxemic conditions, or when testicle removal after death was delayed, the quality of the epididymal semen, and thus the frozen semen, may be compromised.

Another interesting application for frozen epididymal sperm is the possibility to freeze semen from young stallions with no sexual experience that will be submitted to an elective orchiectomy.

The development of new extenders has allowed a significant increase in the quality and consequently fertility of stallion epididymal semen. BotuCrio has been shown to be the best extender to preserve motility and fertility of frozen epididymal sperm providing fertility rates similar to ejaculated frozen sperm.[12]

The epididymal sperm can also be used in such techniques as intracytoplasmatic sperm injection. Consequently, it is advised to freeze some straws with a low number of sperm per straw (eg, 5 million cells) for further use in intracytoplasmatic sperm injection.

Techniques to Recover Semen from the Epididymis

The testicles must be removed from the animal immediately after death or as soon as possible. In this case and in cases of orchiectomy, the duct deferens must be ligated to prevent sperm loss. The testis and attached epididymis must be rinsed with Ringer lactate or saline solution and then packaged in plastic bags or palpation gloves. When the recovery of sperm from the epididymis is not performed immediately, the testis with the epididymis can be stored at 5°C for 24 hours, using the same containers for cooling semen. There are two techniques to obtain sperm from the epididymis: retrograde flushing and flotation technique.

The Retrograde Flushing Technique

Retrograde flushing is the most widely used technique and involves creating pressure within the vas deferens by injecting extender until the epididymal sperm are carried by the extender through the incisions on the tail of the epididymis. The semen may be recovered by washing the tail of the epididymis with the same extender used for cryopreservation (15–20 mL), or by washing with the extender used for centrifugation. We have not observed any differences on postthaw semen quality when flushing straight with the freezing extender or flushing with milk extender and then centrifuging the sample. Flushing with the freezing extender eliminates the centrifugation step. The epididymis is manually dissected to remove the fascia that surround the tail of the epididymis.

Flotation Method

In this technique, the tail of the epididymis is sliced with a scalpel blade in several small pieces to expose the epididymal sperm to the external environment. The tail of the epididymis is then placed in the freezing extender and incubated to allow the sperm to flow into the media for 15 minutes. Then, the sample is filtered using a nylon filter to remove debris. This method can also be performed after the retrograde flush technique to improve the recovery of sperm cells, especially when the epididymis is not completely dissected.

Steps for Cryopreservation of Epididymal Semen

Following the recovery of semen from the tail of the epididymis, the sperm must be concentrated using the previously discussed techniques. When the tail of the epididymis is flushed with the freezing extender, the recovered semen may be frozen directly, without centrifugation. After resuspension with the freezing extender, it is important to wait approximately 10 to 20 minutes to allow sperm to achieve the best motility parameters. Sperm motility usually improves from less than 5% to more than 70% after 10 minutes of incubation in the freezing extender. After the resuspension of the epididymal sperm, the other steps to cryopreserve are the same as described previously for ejaculated semen.

REFERENCES

1. Nath LC, McKinnon AO, Anderson GA. Reproductive efficiency of Thoroughbred and Standardbred horses in north east Victoria. Aust Vet J 2010;88:169–75.
2. Aurich JE, Kuhne A, Hoppe H, et al. Seminal plasma affects membrane integrity and motility of equine spermatozoa after cryopreservation. Theriogenology 1996;46:791–7.
3. Dell'aqua JA, Papa FO, Alvarenga MA, et al. Effect of centrifugation an packing system on sperm parameters of equine frozen semen. Anim Reprod Sci 2001;68:324–5.
4. Loomis PR. Advanced methods for handling and preparation of stallion semen. Vet Clin Equine 2006;22:663–76.
5. Bliss SB, Voge JL, Hayden SS, et al. The impact of cushioned centrifugation protocols on semen quality of stallions. Theriogenology 2012;77:1232–9.

6. Alvarenga MA, Papa FO, Carmo MT, et al. Methods of concentrating stallion semen. J Equine Vet Sci 2012;32:424–9.

7. Alvarenga MA, Papa FO, Landim-Alvarenga FC, et al. Amides as cryoprotectants for freezing stallion semen: a review. Anim Reprod Sci 2005;89:105–13.

8. Metcalf ES. The efficient use of equine cryopreserved semen. Theriogenology 2007;68:423–8.

9. Varner DD, Love CC, Brinsko SP, et al. Semen processing for the subfertile stallion. J Equine Vet Sci 2008;28:677–85.

10. Gutierrez-Cepeda L, Fernandez A, Crespo F, et al. Simple and economic colloidal centrifugation protocols may be incorporated into the clinical equine sperm processing procedure. Anim Reprod Sci 2011;124:85–9.

11. Morrell JM. Stallion sperm selection: past, present, and future trends. J Equine Vet Sci 2012;32:436–40.

12. Monteiro GA, Papa FO, Zahn FS, et al. Cryopreservation and fertility of ejaculated and epididymal stallion sperm. Anim Reprod Sci 2011;127:197–201.

Modern Techniques for Semen Evaluation

Charles C. Love, DVM, PhD

KEYWORDS

- Semen • Semen evaluation • Fertility • Stallion • Breeding

KEY POINTS

- The semen evaluation should be performed as part of a complete breeding soundness evaluation.
- The effect of mare and management factors should be taken into account when the results of the semen evaluation are interpreted.
- Understand how to use the tests and the limitations of each test.
- Test limitations can have a profound effect on the interpretation of the results.
- Test results should be interpreted accounting for the influence nonstallion factors may have on the presenting complaint (eg, subfertility).

INTRODUCTION

The evaluation of stallion semen is an integral part of evaluating horse subfertility and determining a stallions potential as a breeding prospect. Although semen evaluation is an important part of a stallion's breeding potential, good sperm quality is necessary, but not sufficient, for fertility. This concept is important because a semen evaluation is often performed as a separate "stand-alone test" with little knowledge of the limitations that may be imposed by the mare or management. In general, there are 3 factors that affect fertility: the stallion, the mare, and management (ie, human component). Often when the clinician is presented with inadequate fertility the stallion or the mare are assumed to be the source of the problem. Currently, there are many semen tests, most of which are sperm quality tests. Coincidental with the application of a sperm test the clinician should interpret the results of the test to the client. In general, sperm quality tests tend to be correlated with other sperm quality tests (ie, if one is "good" others are also "good") and oftentimes the clinician and client may interpret additional testing as providing little value. However, these tests can provide unique information about individual stallion that is not obvious from results of other tests.

In general, there are 2 circumstances when a semen evaluation is performed (1) as a stand-alone test when the fertility of the stallion is in question owing to poor fertility

Department of Large Animal Clinical Sciences, College of Veterinary Medicine, Texas A&M University, College Station, TX 77843, USA
E-mail address: clove@cvm.tamu.edu

Vet Clin Equine 32 (2016) 531–546
http://dx.doi.org/10.1016/j.cveq.2016.07.006
0749-0739/16/© 2016 Elsevier Inc. All rights reserved.

outcome and (2) to determine a stallions potential fertility stallions may or may not have a prior breeding history.

In all species, there is a constant pursuit of the holy grail of sperm quality tests. Essentially, a single test, that when applied to a semen sample, explains/predicts stallion fertility. This is a naïve pursuit; as veterinary clinicians, we understand implicitly that horse fertility is composed of much more than sperm quality. In addition, there are many self-imposed limitations to how the evaluation of sperm quality is performed as well as what tests are used and how they are interpreted. Understanding these limitations is critical as the clinician is required not just to perform the test but to interpret the results.

Although there have been many new "sperm tests" introduced relatively recently, few are validated regarding their relationship to fertility. The clinician should be cautious in promoting tests unless interpretation of the results relative to fertility can be presented to the client.

SPERM MOTILITY

Sperm motility is, historically, the most common test of sperm quality, primarily because of the ease of evaluation under a variety of conditions. Biologically, the ability of a sperm to be motile is certainly necessary for fertility, but the type and quality of motility can be affected by the conditions (eg, hot, cold, osmotic changes) under which the test is determined. Therefore, the sperm motility test should be conducted under well-controlled conditions, such that the results reflect the inherent sperm quality of the stallion tested and not iatrogenic influences. If these conditions cannot be accommodated, then the results should be interpreted accordingly. Ideally, sperm motility should be tested using a phase-contrast microscope with both ×20 and ×40 objectives such that the final magnification should be ×200 and ×400, respectively. The microscope should be equipped with a warm stage that can be adjusted to 37°C. These magnification levels allow a clear visualization of a low- and high-power view of the sperm sample. Light microscopy should be avoided because clear visualization (ie, the ability of the eye to identify immotile sperm), especially at a low magnification, may be insufficient. The inability to identify immotile sperm may result in a falsely high motility value.

Microscopically, sperm motility is evaluated under a variety of conditions, all of which can result in a value that may inaccurately reflect stallions inherent sperm quality. The magnification (eg, ×100–×1000), type of microscope (eg, light, phase contrast), working conditions (eg, heated stage, ambient temperature), evaluator experience, as well as unknown influences that may be toxic to sperm, are just a few examples of factors unrelated to the intrinsic sperm motility of the stallion. Therefore, the clinician should be cautious about the interpretation of sperm motility results when they seem to be inconsistent with other clinical findings.

Adding to the subjectivity of evaluating sperm motility are the different types of sperm motility evaluated, which include total motility (TMOT) and progressive motility (PMOT). Of these 2, PMOT is the most problematic. Sperm that are "progressive" are considered to be moving in a relatively straight forward motion and are assumed to be more "fertile." Historically, sperm progressivity is assumed to imply normality, whereas other nonprogressive sperm are considered pathologic. As the evaluation of sperm quality has evolved and additional sperm quality tests have been introduced, it has become clear that the measurement of progressive sperm motility is outdated. The factors mentioned that lead to variation are particularly worrisome when PMOT is evaluated. These artifactual factors have the potential to render a low PMOT value in a sample from a fertile stallion. This requires the clinician to interpret these low PMOT samples as limited in their fertility potential, which in turn may result in a failed breeding contract, sale of the stallion, and animosity between the parties involved in the transaction. Although these kinds of outcomes may have been unavoidable in the past, the increased knowledge and number of high-quality sperm tests has provided the clinician with the ability to verify whether an apparently poor quality sperm sample is indeed poor or simply an artifact.

Computer-assisted sperm analyzers are available and provide a more objective method, in most cases, to evaluate sperm motility. These systems provide a variety of motility values, including TMOT, velocity values, and compound measures such as PMOT, straightness, and linearity. The compound measures vary based on thresholds set by the operator. Interestingly, PMOT like the other compound measures can be set to be as high or low as the operator desires, because there is no accepted "standard" for PMOT. Computer-assisted sperm analyzer systems are particularly useful in the research arena because of the objectivity and repeatability of the measures evaluated.

SEMEN VOLUME

The measurement of semen volume is a fundamental measure that, in combination with sperm concentration, determines the total number of sperm ejaculated by the stallion. Semen volume may have considerable variation owing to the measurement technique. Sperm numbers can be reduced by losses in the artificial vagina[1] or by the type of measuring device (**Fig. 1**). Often, volume is measured in wide mouthed cups with measure graduations that are far apart, making volume measurement an approximation rather than an accurate result. Ideally, it is recommended to measure volume by weighing the sample or using a graduated cylinder. The former technique has the advantage of not requiring the removal of the semen volume from the collection bag to another container, which, in the process results in sperm loss unless the collection container is rinsed with semen extender.

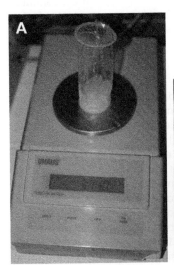
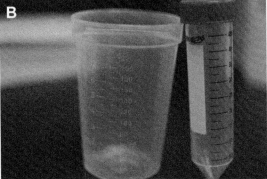

Fig. 1. Different methods of measuring semen volume. (*A*) Digital scale with a semen collection receptacle (baby bottle liner). (*B*) Wide-mouthed plastic cup and 50-mL polystyrene tube.

SPERM CONCENTRATION

The measurement of sperm concentration, similar to semen volume, is a partial measure that allows the calculation of total sperm number. The only direct measure (ie, actually visualizing sperm) of sperm concentration is hemacytometry.[2] Owing to time and inconvenience, this technique has been displaced by spectrophotometric devices that measure the change in fluid opacity. These techniques make the assumption that the change in opacity from the clear control sample to the unknown semen sample is only a result of added sperm. This assumption is incorrect and in certain circumstances, the nonsperm material, will dramatically inflate the number of sperm measured. For example, seminal plasma alone imparts a level of opacity that can result in a reading of 10 to 20 million sperm/mL or higher depending on the level of contamination with epithelial cells (ie, smegma). Therefore, perhaps the most important reason for thoroughly washing a stallion's penis is to ensure that there is minimal epithelial cell contamination. The opacity of seminal plasma becomes more important the lower the actual sperm concentration. Often semen with a low concentration also has a higher volume, in which case the ratio of seminal plasma and actual sperm concentration may approach 1 (50/50 v/v). This example would result in a doubling of the expected sperm number from that ejaculate and the inseminate would actually contain only 50% of the expected sperm number. This may be an unrecognized source of reduced fertility when artificial insemination is used.

Recently, an alternative more accurate method of measuring sperm concentration and sperm viability has become available. The Nucleocounter (NC [NucleoCounter SP-100; ChemoMetec A/S, Allerød, Denmark]) is a fluorescent-based machine that uses propidium iodide (PI), a DNA-specific fluorescent probe that attaches to sperm DNA. This technique has the ability to discern sperm and nonsperm material. The NC is also able to evaluate sperm concentration and viability in extended semen not just raw semen. Therefore, frozen–thawed and cool-shipped semen can be evaluated to determine the accuracy of the semen "dose." These measures cannot be performed in the spectrophotometric machines because the particulate matter of extender interfere with light transmission causing a false high sperm concentration value. The clinician, should however be cautious, because semen contamination with somatic DNA fragments the size of sperm will also stain with the PI and "cross-react," resulting in an inflated sperm number.

MORPHOLOGIC FEATURES

The evaluation of sperm morphologic features identifies the shape of normal and abnormal sperm forms. It can be performed using several different preparation methods including a background stain such as eosin–nigrosin (EN) or a wet mount technique in which the semen sample is fixed in a buffered formol saline solution. The EN technique has the advantage of also evaluating viability and being a quicker and simpler technique requiring only a light microscope and low magnification. The EN technique has the potential to induce artifactual morphologic changes (eg, bent tails, detached heads) owing to composition changes in the stain or preparation error. In addition, the EN technique, owing to the lesser quality of the image, may result in the clinician missing subtle, but fertility limiting abnormalities such as abnormal midpieces. The buffered formol saline technique is usually performed at a magnification of ×1000 using either phase-contrast or differential interference microscopy, techniques that provide enhanced resolution compared with light microscopy. Compared with other sperm quality assays such as motility and viability, samples prepared for sperm morphology are not time dependent, but can be fixed at a remote location and then evaluated at a later time at a referral laboratory.

The evaluation of sperm morphology is the only test that is a reflection of the stallion's intrinsic sperm quality. Our laboratory has maintained a similar classification system as the stallion breeding soundness evaluation manual.[3] In addition to the percent normal sperm, the types of abnormalities include abnormal acrosomes, heads, and midpieces; proximal and distal droplets; detached normal heads; bent midpieces and tails; coiled tails; and premature germ cells (**Fig. 2**). Identifying specific abnormalities rather than packaging abnormalities into large categories such as primary/secondary or major/minor classification systems is preferred because individual sperm morphogenetic features can aid in the diagnosis, prognosis, and treatment of certain conditions. Some abnormalities are associated with transient conditions such as sperm accumulation (eg, detached abnormal heads, hairpin tail, distal droplets), whereas others are associated with testicular dysfunction (abnormal heads and midpieces, coiled tails, and premature germ cells). In addition, certain abnormalities, when they occur together in sufficient numbers, tend to be associated with a reduction in fertility (Refs.[4–7]; see **Tables 3** and **5**).

FLOW CYTOMETRIC ASSAYS

Recently, there has been an explosion of flow cytometric assays available for the evaluation of sperm characteristics. These assays are usually applied to sperm after they have been validated and marketed for somatic cells. Although sperm have many of the same physiologic features of somatic cells, they are nevertheless very different cells. Therefore, the protocols and conclusions that are drawn from somatic cell studies may be inadequate when applied to sperm. If assays are to be applied to sperm of any species, it is essential that the tests be validated for sperm and for that species. From a clinical perspective, we are interested in whether these tests can aid our understanding of fertility, whether they are independent of other tests, and not just describe a physiologic somatic cell function that also happens to occur in sperm. This is a relatively high standard, because determining the relationship between a sperm function test to fertility is time consuming and expensive.

SPERM CHROMATIN STRUCTURE ASSAY

This assay was introduced by Don Evenson as a measure of the susceptibility of sperm DNA to denature after a short incubation period in a low pH solution.[8] This concept relies on the hypothesis that sperm DNA, which responds to a low pH environment by exhibiting a greater degree of denaturation, is less stable, and therefore may result in reduced fertility compared with more stable sperm DNA. The assay measures this loss of DNA stability by determining the fluorescent ratio of single (ie, denatured DNA) to double-stranded DNA (native) in the sperm head. The fluorescent dye, acridine orange, fluoresces green when it attaches to double-stranded DNA and red-orange when attached to single-stranded DNA. Individual sperm, therefore, exhibit both green and red fluorescence, which the flow cytometer detects and presents as a 2-dimensional image (**Fig. 3**). The main (normal) population is represented as an elliptical population on the left side of the screen, and the sperm with more single-stranded DNA (ie, more red fluorescence) are to the right of this population. The population in which sperm have more single-stranded DNA is termed the percent of cells outside the main population (% COMP-$_{\alpha t}$) or DNA index. The % COMP-$_{\alpha t}$ is the most common value reported and represents only those sperm that are different from the main population. This assumes that the main population is normal. There, are

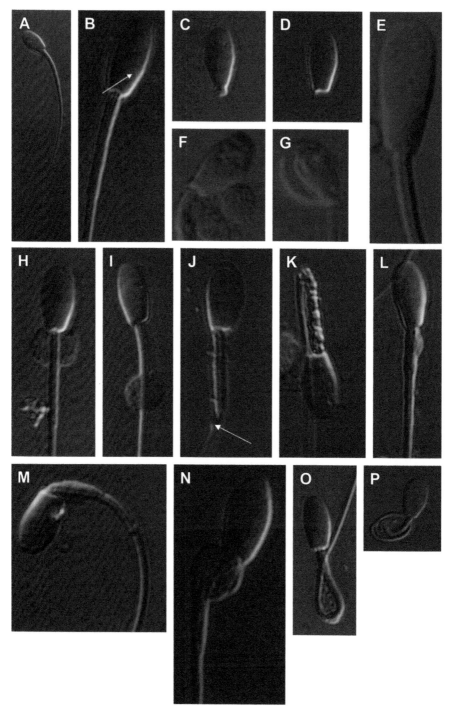

Fig. 2. Morphologic sperm shapes. (*A*) Normal. Notice the small crater. This is considered normal and occurs in a high percentage of sperm from fertile stallions. (*B*) Raised acrosome (*arrow*). Commonly results from freeze–thaw damage and cooled storage.

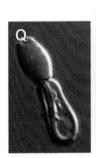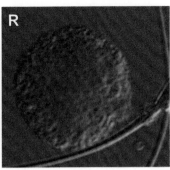

Fig. 2. (*continued*).

however, instances when the whole sperm population has shifted (ie, essentially 100% COMP). This change may only be detected if the average value for all the sperm is determined. The shift in the whole population is measured by the Mean-$_{\alpha t}$ and Mode-$_{\alpha t}$. In addition, the standard deviation (SD-$_{\alpha t}$), is also measured and reflects the degree of single-stranded DNA of individual sperm. In stallions, increases in the Mean-$_{\alpha t}$ and COMP-$_{\alpha t}$ are the endpoints associated with a decrease in fertility (Refs.[7,9]; **Table 1**; see **Table 6**). The assay can measure the DNA quality of both native sperm DNA and the change in the quality of DNA from aged sperm after cool storage.[10]

SPERM VIABILITY

Sperm viability is a generic term that refers to the overall health of the sperm; however, when sperm viability is measured using stains or fluorescent probes it refers to the ability of these stains or probes to penetrate a damaged or intact sperm membrane. Historically, the most common sperm stain used in theriogenology is the EN stain. It is used as a background stain to highlight the pale appearing viable sperm. It also has the property that it will penetrate a damaged membrane and color the sperm a pale red color (**Fig. 4**).

The Nucleocounter (NC) uses PI, a fluorescent stain that only penetrates damaged membranes and binds to DNA to evaluate viability. Two semen samples must be evaluated. The first evaluates sperm concentration and exposes the sperm to a detergent solution that damages the membranes of all the sperm, thus allowing penetration of the PI into all of the sperm. The second sample uses a physiologic solution (eg, phosphate-buffered saline) that maintains the integrity of those native sperm with intact membranes and stains only sperm with inherently damaged sperm membranes. The results of the second sample are subtracted from the first sample to determine the percent viability.

(*C*) Morphologically normal detached head. (*D*) Morphologically abnormal detached head. Notice damaged acrosome. (*E–G*) Abnormal head shapes. (*H*) Proximal droplet. (*I*) Distal droplet. Abnormal midpieces. (*J*) Roughened midpiece with segmental aplasia (*arrow*). (*K*) Swollen midpiece characteristic of damage after cooling or freeze–thaw. (*L, M*) Swollen midpiece. (*N*) Malformed midpiece, not to be confused with a proximal droplet. (*O*) Bent midpiece (also termed hairpin/bent tail). (*P, Q*) Coiled tail, (*R*) Premature germ cell.

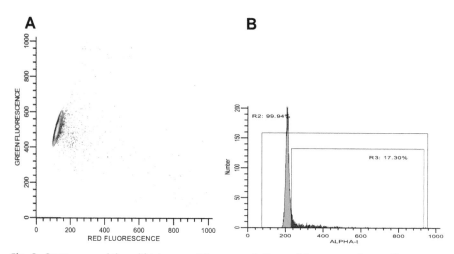

Fig. 3. Scattergram (*A*) and histogram (*B*) representations of the sperm chromatin structure assay results. (*A*) Raw data obtained from the flow cytometer. The main population is represented as the elliptical region to the left and the percent of cells outside the main population (% COMP) is represented by the purple cells to the right of the main population. Both cell populations can be represented in histogram form in *B*. In this case the % COMP is 17.3%.

There are many potential flow cytometric based viability assays. Two common assays use a combination of SYBR-14 and PI or pea lectin (*Pisum sativum*) and PI. The SYBR-14/PI combination is commercially available as a kit (Molecular Probes LIVE/DEAD Sperm Viability Kit, Molecular Probes, Eugene, OR). The SYBR-14 stain penetrates both intact and damaged sperm membranes and fluoresces green/yellow, whereas the PI will only penetrate a damaged membrane, but will overwhelm the fluorescence of the SYBR-14 and stain the sperm red. Both of these stains bind to DNA (**Fig. 5**).

In unfixed samples, the *Pisum sativum*/PI stain positively identifies sperm with damaged acrosomes and sperm membranes, but only identifies viable and acrosomes-intact sperm by their lack of stain uptake. This assay has the advantage of evaluating acrosome status, but may be limited in some instances because viable sperm are identified by a lack of stain uptake rather than stain acquisition and relies on the assumption that all objects that do not acquire the PI stain are viable (**Figs. 6 and 7**).

LONGEVITY OF SPERM QUALITY

Since the introduction of cool-shipped semen, evaluation of the ability of a sperm sample to survive for a period of time (usually 24 hours) has become more relevant. All of the sperm quality tests described can be used to evaluate the longevity of sperm quality except morphology.

EVALUATION OF COOL-SHIPPED SEMEN

Overall, the fertility of stored, cool-shipped stallion semen is less than fresh semen inseminated immediately after collection.[11,12] Causes for this difference include the need for better mare management (ie, synchronization of ovulation and insemination), semen processing, and identification of stallions whose semen may require additional

Table 1
Sperm parameter, threshold value, and embryo recovery

Sperm Parameter	Threshold[a]	Embryo Recovery Rate[b]		Sperm Quality Values[c]	
		Average	High	Average	High
Total sperm motility (%)	$\geq$65	93/174 (53)	153/230 (67)	50 $\pm$ 11 (5–60)	69 $\pm$ 5 (65–85)
Progressively sperm motility (%)	$\geq$45	57/107 (53)	189/287 (64)	36 $\pm$ 11 (0–45)	59 $\pm$ 6 (50–75)
Viable sperm (%)	$\geq$71	70/138 (51)	178/269 (66)	56 $\pm$ 18 (0–71)	80 $\pm$ 5 (71–92)
Morphologically normal (%)	$\geq$47	46/97 (47)	170/269 (63)	35 $\pm$ 10 (5–46)	64 $\pm$ 10 (47–88)
Total sperm number (billions)	$\geq$1.14	64/129 (50)	181/272 (67)	0.78 $\pm$ 0.22 (0.20–1.12)	1.91 $\pm$ 0.86 (1.14–6.67)
Total motile sperm (billions)	<0.60	53/114 (46)	189/283 (67)	0.4 $\pm$ 0.1 (0.03–0.6)	1.2 $\pm$ 0.6 (0.6–5.3)
Total morphologically normal (billions)	<0.94	117/222 (53)	84/112 (75)	0.57 $\pm$ 0.23 (0.06–0.94)	1.4 $\pm$ 0.63 (0.94–4.20)
Total progressively motile sperm (billions)	<0.55	61/129 (47)	181/268 (68)	0.4 $\pm$ 0.2 (0.01–0.5)	1.1 $\pm$ 0.5 (0.5–4.7)
Sperm concentration (mil/mL)	$\geq$31.6	72/141 (51)	182/277 (66)	22 $\pm$ 6 (4–32)	60 $\pm$ 48 (32–482)
Total viable sperm (billion)	<0.74	59/120 (49)	186/280 (66)	0.5 $\pm$ 0.2 (0.07–0.7)	1.4 $\pm$ 0.7 (0.8–5.6)
Total progressively motile viable sperm (billion)	<0.32	39/95 (41)	203/301 (67)	0.2 $\pm$ 0.1 (0–0.3)	0.8 $\pm$ 0.4 (0.3–3.8)
Total motile morphologically normal sperm (billion)	$\leq$0.37	65/121 (54)	134/210 (64)	0.2 $\pm$ 0.1 (.01–0.4)	0.7 $\pm$ 0.4 (0.4–3.4)
% COMP$_{\alpha t}$	$\geq$26.8	14/33 (42)	147/236 (62)	33 $\pm$ 13 (27–72)	13 $\pm$ 5 (4–27)
Mean$_{\alpha t}$	$\leq$253	39/85 (46)	122/184 (66)	273 $\pm$ 22 (254–374)	233 $\pm$ 14 (186–254)
Mode$_{\alpha t}$	>233	44/93 (47)	117/175 (67)	244 $\pm$ 16 (233–374)	216 $\pm$ 13 (165–232)

[a] Threshold value that separates the average and high fertility groups.
[b] Embryos recovered/total attempts (% recovery rate). Between columns all rates are different at the $P<.05$ level.
[c] Represents mean $\pm$ standard deviation (range) sperm quality value for the average and high fertility groups. Between columns all rates are different.

From Love CC, Noble JK, Standridge SA, et al. The relationship between sperm quality in cool-shipped semen and embryo recovery rate in horses. Theriogenology 2015;84:1590; with permission.

processing (ie, centrifugation) before cooling and shipment. A common concern with cool-shipped sperm is low sperm motility and can result from either inherently poor sperm quality that originates from inadequate semen handling and processing after semen collection (ie, iatrogenic).

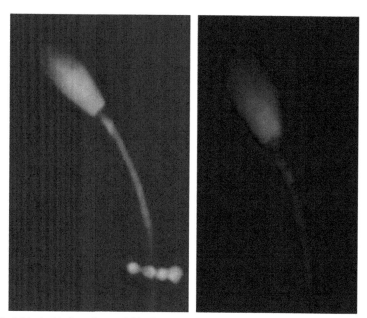

Fig. 4. A viable (*white*) and nonviable (*pink*) sperm head after eosin–nigrosin staining.

Diagnostically, this is a challenge to the clinician because the consequences may not only affect fertility, but client satisfaction. As with all evaluations of sperm quality, it is critical to perform a complete evaluation and not rely on a single sperm quality test. In the case of low sperm motility, complete testing is usually diagnostic. Sperm morphology will identify those samples with inherently poor sperm quality as well as those samples with a high percent of normal sperm yet low motility. In the latter

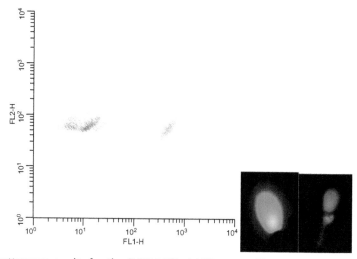

Fig. 5. Scattergram results for the SYBR-14/PI viability assay. The green population represents viable sperm (SYBR-14 positive); the red population represents the propidium iodide (PI) nonviable population; the population between the 2 represents transitional sperm that are acquiring PI (ie, becoming nonviable).

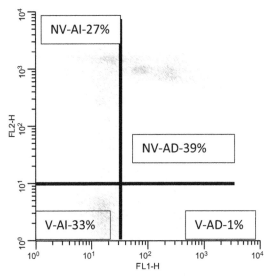

Fig. 6. Scattergram representing viability (ie, membrane intactness) and acrosomal membrane intactness. Regions: NV-AD, nonviable/acrosome damaged; NV-AI, nonviable/acrosome intact; V-AD, viable/acrosome damaged; V-AI; viable/acrosome intact.

case, this suggests that the semen sample has been altered after collection. In the face of a high percent of normal sperm, low sperm motility, however, does not mean that the sample is poor quality. Sperm samples that are initially of high motility may lose motility yet retain viability. This is commonly caused by a high percent (ie, >15%–20%) of seminal plasma in the extended cool-shipped sample.[13] These low motility/high viability samples can be fertile[14] and should therefore not be discarded, but should be inseminated. This has been appreciated anecdotally since the introduction of cooled-shipped semen based on reports of stallions whose "semen does not ship well," but who have good fertility. The clinician should not assume that samples of low motility are poor quality without also measuring the viability and morphology of the sample.

INTERPRETATION

A thorough interpretation of a semen evaluation should account for the role of the mare and management. The evaluation should include measurement of sperm

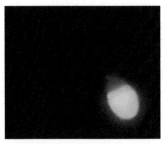

Fig. 7. A *Pisum sativum*/propidium iodide stained sperm that identifies a damaged/reacted acrosome and nonviable sperm membrane, respectively.

concentration, semen volume, initial sperm motility, longevity of sperm motility, morphology, and viability. These tests can be supplemented with additional testing such as the sperm chromatin structure assay.

The clinician should avoid dogmatic conclusions based on cutoff values from individual tests (ie, PMOT < 60% is abnormal), but rather include the results of multiple tests to determine whether the apparently low value of one test is consistent with the levels of the other tests. The effect of an incorrect diagnosis, in which a result from a single sperm quality test is reported as "poor," can have long-term economic implications for a stallion's breeding potential and his future reputation.

For example, a stallion may exhibit "normal" sperm motility even though the percent of morphologically normal sperm may be low and fertility may be reduced. Most abnormalities may exhibit motility (eg, abnormal heads and midpieces; proximal and distal droplets; bent tails and midpieces) and many may also be viable (abnormal heads and midpieces; proximal and distal droplets; bent tails and midpieces as well as coiled tails). Therefore, if the clinician relies solely on an individual sperm test, such as motility or viability to render an opinion on a stallion's sperm quality, it is possible that important fertility-limiting morphologic features may be missed even though motility and viability values are "normal."

Threshold sperm quality values that differentiate ejaculates of high and average fertility are reported in **Table 1**. These were samples from commercial stallions and stallions with overt subfertility were not included. Therefore, it is likely that sperm quality values below those reported may be associated with lesser fertility. Generally, in this study embryo recovery rate for average and high fertility was approximately 50% and 65%, respectively.

Results of another study (**Tables 2–5**) evaluated sperm motility and morphology and their relationship to the seasonal pregnancy rate (SPR), which was divided

Table 2
Stallion sperm motility variables for the seasonal pregnancy rate from mares

	1 (n = 22)	2 (n = 11)
Seasonal pregnancy rate (%)	90 ± 6 (79–100)	58 ± 21 (12–77)
Pregnant/cycle (%)	62 ± 16 (36–100)	41 ± 17 (8–66)
Pregnant/first cycle (%)	62 ± 22 (0–100)	48 ± 17 (14–80)
Total motility (%)[a]	78 ± 12 (44–92)	68 ± 20 (18–88)
Progressive motility (%)	72 ± 12 (43–88)	63 ± 20 (16–84)
Rapid (%)	69 ± 12 (41–87)	60 ± 20 (13–84)
Moderate (%)	3 ± 2 (1–8)	3 ± 1 (2–6)
Slow (%)	5 ± 2 (1–11)	4 ± 1 (2–6)
Anticrit	0.81 ± 0.44 (0–2)	0.73 ± 0.7 (0–2.3)
Critical value	88 ± 5 (74–95)	87 ± 6 (73–94)
Linearity	77 ± 4 (69–84)	76 ± 5 (67–82)
Path velocity (μ/s)	193 ± 23 (157–241)	178 ± 27 (104–199)
Progressive velocity (μ/s)[b]	173 ± 19 (143–208)	157 ± 25 (88–183)

Seasonal pregnancy rate groups: group 1, ≥78% and ≤100%; group 2, ≥0% and <78%.
  Values are presented as means ± standard deviation (range).
  [a] P = .08.
  [b] P = .06.
  From Love CC. Relationship between sperm motility, morphology and the fertility of stallions. Theriogenology 2011;76:550; with permission.

Table 3
Stallion sperm morphology variables for the seasonal pregnancy rate from mares

Morphology Variables	1 (n = 56)	2 (n = 19)
Normal	51 ± 18 (11–85)	43 ± 23 (4–75)
Abnormal heads	12 ± 10 (0–45)	14 ± 10 (1–43)
Detached heads	2 ± 2 (0–10)	4 ± 10 (1–44)
Proximal droplets	19 ± 15 (2–60)	23 ± 17 (8–70)
Distal droplets	7 ± 6 (0–28)	5 ± 5 (0–17)
Bent midpieces	0.23 ± 0.62 (0–4)	1 ± 4 (0–17)
General midpiece abnormality	7 ± 6 (1–29)	8 ± 6 (3–26)
Hairpin tail	4 ± 4 (0–16)	5 ± 6 (0–20)
Coiled tail[a]	2 ± 2 (0–11)	4 ± 4 (0–14)
Premature germ cell	1.5 ± 1.7 (0–8)	1.3 ± 2.1 (0–7)

Seasonal pregnancy rate groups: group 1, ≥78% and ≤100%; group 2, ≥ 0% and <78%.
Values are presented as means ± standard deviation (range).
[a] $P = .02$.
From Love CC. Relationship between sperm motility, morphology and the fertility of stallions. Theriogenology 2011;76:550; with permission.

Table 4
Stallion sperm motility variables for the percent mares pregnant/cycle

	1 (n = 8)	2 (n = 20)	3 (n = 4)
Seasonal pregnancy rate (%)	97 ± 4 (90–100)	86 ± 10 (50–100)	61 ± 29 (12–100)
Pregnant/cycle (%)	91 ± 10 (75–100)	56 ± 6 (45–74)	32 ± 13 (8–45)
Pregnant/first cycle (%)	91 ± 10 (75–100)	58 ± 16 (0–88)	34 ± 14 (0–50)
Total motility (%)[a]	83 ± 5 (76–91)[a]	76 ± 12 (44–92)[a]	48 ± 21 (18–66)[b]
Progressive motility (%)[b]	77 ± 6 (64–85)[a]	71 ± 12 (43–88)[a]	44 ± 20 (16–63)[b]
Rapid (%)[c]	74 ± 9 (57–83)[a]	68 ± 12 (41–88)[a]	42 ± 20 (13–60)[b]
Moderate (%)	4 ± 2 (2–8)	3 ± 1 (1–6)	3 ± 0.2 (2–3)
Slow (%)	6 ± 3 (2–11)	4 ± 2 (1–9)	4 ± 1 (2–6)
Anticrit	0.9 ± 0.7 (0–2)	0.8 ± 0.3 (0.3–1.3)	0.6 ± 1.3 (0–2.3)
Critical value[d]	87 ± 7 (74–95)[a]	89 ± 4 (81–95)[a]	83 ± 7 (73–90)[b]
Linearity	77 ± 3 (74–84)	77 ± 4 (67–82)	74 ± 4 (69–78)
Path velocity (μ/s)[e]	196 ± 26 (163–230)[a]	190 ± 19 (157–241)[a]	162 ± 41 (104–194)[b]
Progressive velocity (μ/s)[f]	174 ± 20 (146–207)[a]	171 ± 17 (143–208)[a]	139 ± 34 (88–166)[b]

Percent pregnant/cycle groups: group 1, ≥76% and ≤100%; group 2, ≥ 46% and <76%; group 3, ≥ 0% and <46%.
Values are presented as means ± standard deviation (range).
[a] $P<.0001$.
[b] $P<.001$.
[c] $P<.0002$.
[d] $P<.04$.
[e] $P<.04$.
[f] $P<.008$.
From Love CC. Relationship between sperm motility, morphology and the fertility of stallions. Theriogenology 2011;76:551; with permission.

Table 5
Stallion sperm morphology variables for the percent mares pregnant/cycle

Morphology Variables	1 (n = 11)	2 (n = 49)	3 (n = 13)
Normal[a]	67 ± 8 (50–76)[a]	48 ± 15 (17–83)[b]	41 ± 27 (7–85)[b]
Abnormal heads	9 ± 6 (1–22)	12 ± 9 (0–45)	17 ± 13 (1–43)
Detached heads[b]	2 ± 2 (1–8)[a]	2 ± 2 (1–10)[a]	6 ± 11 (0–44)[b]
Proximal droplets[c]	8 ± 3 (5–14)[a]	20 ± 14 (2–51)[b]	25 ± 18 (4–60)[b]
Distal droplets[d]	6 ± 4 (2–16)[a]	8 ± 7 (0–28)[a]	2 ± 2 (1–7)[b]
Bent midpieces	1 ± 1 (0–4)	0.2 ± 0.4 (0–1)	1 ± 5 (0–17)
General midpiece abnormality[e]	6 ± 4 (1–14)[a]	7 ± 6 (1–29)[ab]	10 ± 6 (2–26)[b]
Hairpin tail	4 ± 3 (0–9)	4 ± 4 (0–16)	5 ± 6 (0–20)
Coiled tail[f]	1 ± 1 (0–3)[a]	2 ± 2 (0–7)[a]	5 ± 5 (0–14)[b]
Premature germ cell	1 ± 2 (0–6)	1 ± 2 (0–8)	2 ± 2 (0–7)

Percent pregnant/cycle groups: Group 1, ≥76% and ≤100%; Group 2, ≥46% and <76%; Group 3, ≥0% and <46%.
  Values are presented as means ± standard deviation (range).
  [a] $P<.002$.
  [b] $P<.03$.
  [c] $P<.0008$.
  [d] $P<.03$.
  [e] $P<.03$.
  [f] $P<.04$.
From Love CC. Relationship between sperm motility, morphology and the fertility of stallions. Theriogenology 2011;76:551; with permission.

into 2 classes (>78% or <78%) and pregnancy rate per cycle (PRC), which was divided into 3 classes (>76%; >46% and <76; and <46%). Sperm motility values and most morphologic values were unable to differentiate SPR rate classes; however, these same measures of sperm quality were able to identify differences in PRC classes. These results are unlikely owing to the inadequacy of the tests themselves, but rather the increased sensitivity of the method used to measure fertility (ie, PRC > SPR).

In the same study, sperm motility values discriminate the lowest PRC level from the high and average levels, but values between the high and average levels are similar. In contrast, the percent of morphologically normal sperm are similar between the average and low PRC levels, but higher in the high PRC group. This is useful diagnostically and suggests that sperm motility (TMOT) may be a better test to identify stallions of lesser fertility. A reduction in fertility is not noticed until TMOT reaches a level of about 50% (see **Tables 1** and **4**).

The percent of morphologically normal sperm, in contrast, does not discriminate low and average levels of PRC. This result, however, can be explained partially by the types of abnormalities identified in the low and average PRC groups (see **Table 5**). The low PRC group has more abnormalities associated with testes dysfunction (abnormal head and midpieces, detached heads, and coiled tails), whereas the average PRC group has fewer of those abnormalities and more distal droplets. Interestingly, the level of proximal droplets is similar and relatively high between the average and low PRC groups compared with the high PRC group. Anecdotally, we observe that proximal droplets increase with age and when they reach very high levels (80%–90%), they can be associated with a dramatic decrease in fertility.

Fertility Parameter and Sperm Chromatin Structure Assay Variable	Fertility Group 1	2	3
SPR	90 ± 6 (79–100)	58 ± 21 (12–77)	NA
$\quad$ Mean$_{\alpha t}$[5]	232 ± 16 (203–297)	241 ± 23 (222–296)	NA
$\quad$ SD$_{\alpha t}$	85 ± 22 (50–149)	90 ± 26 (55–171)	NA
$\quad$ COMP$_{\alpha t}$[3]	16 ± 8 (4–38)[a]	23 ± 13 (9–52)[b]	NA
FCP	89 ± 9 (78–100)	58 ± 7 (46–75)	25 ± 18 (0–45)
$\quad$ Mean$_{\alpha t}$	227 ± 9 (213–243)	233 ± 16 (208–297)	237 ± 21 (203–281)
$\quad$ SD$_{\alpha t}$[4]	73 ± 11 (54–96)	89 ± 21 (50–149)	94 ± 30 (55–171)
$\quad$ COMP$_{\alpha t}$[2]	12 ± 5 (4–28)[a]	17 ± 7 (6–38)[b]	25 ± 13 (5–52)[c]
PC	91 ± 10 (75–100)	56 ± 6 (45–74)	32 ± 13 (8–45)
$\quad$ Mean$_{\alpha t}$[4]	229 ± 11 (213–243)[a]	233 ± 15 (206–297)[a]	248 ± 27 (203–296)[b]
$\quad$ SD$_{\alpha t}$	76 ± 12 (62–96)	87 ± 22 (50–149)	97 ± 30 (55–171)
$\quad$ COMP$_{\alpha t}$[1]	13 ± 6 (7–28)[a]	17 ± 7 (4–38)[a]	27 ± 14 (5–52)[b]

Fertility groups: seasonal pregnancy rate (SPR)—group 1, SPR >80%, group 2, SPR <80%; first cycle pregnancy rate (FCP)—group 1, FCP >75%, group 2, FCP <75% and >45%, group 3, FCP <45%; overall cycles per pregnancy (PC)—group 1, PC >75%, group 2, PC <75% and >45%, group 3, PC <45%.
Values are presented as mean ± standard deviation (range).
Letters within rows are different based on the following significance levels: 1, $P<.0001$; 2, $P<.001$; 3, $P<.004$; 4, $P<.01$; 5, $P<.06$.
From Love CC, Kenney RM. The relationship of increased susceptibility of sperm DNA to denaturation and fertility in the stallion. Theriogenology 1998;50:962; with permission.

In a separate publication (**Table 6**) using the same semen samples, the sperm chromatin structure assay was able to discriminate differences in both the SPR and PRC.

The results in **Tables 2–6** do not report the total sperm number (dose) inseminated and therefore it is possible that some "lower" quality ejaculates are compensated by using higher sperm numbers. Nevertheless, both of these studies suggest that ejaculates with high sperm quality should result in high fertility and ejaculates of lesser quality have the potential for reduced fertility. The fertility of any ejaculate has the potential to be modified, either up or down, based on the quality of semen management or mare reproductive quality.

"High" sperm motility is usually associated with good fertility[4,7,12,15] (see **Tables 1, 2, and 4**), except in some unusual cases. The most extreme example are those stallions whose acrosomes do not react after stimulation with calcium ionosphere (A23187).[16,17] These individuals tend to be characterized by excellent overall sperm quality, regardless of the sperm test measured.

The clinician should also beware that many morphologic abnormalities are motile, such as abnormal heads and midpieces, proximal and distal droplets, and hairpin tails (swim backward). Interestingly, proximal droplets may exhibit better longevity of sperm motility than the "normal" sperm population. Awareness of these limitations in the appearance of "good motility" have become particularly relevant as use of cooled and frozen-thawed sperm has become more widespread nationally and internationally. This may explain, in part, why some samples with "good" sperm motility do not result in a commensurate level of fertility.

REFERENCES

1. Pickett BW, Gebauer MR, Seidel GE, et al. Reproductive physiology of the stallion: spermatozoal losses in the collection equipment and gel. J Am Vet Med Assoc 1974;165:708–10.
2. Rigby SL, Varner DD, Thompson JA, et al. Measurement of sperm concentration in stallion ejaculates using photometric or direct sperm enumeration techniques. In: Proceedings 47th Annual American Association of Equine Practitioners. 2001. p. 236–8.
3. Kenney RM, Hurtgen J, Pierson R, et al. Theriogenology and the equine part II: the stallion. In: Society for Theriogenology Manual for clinical fertility evaluation of the stallion. 1983.
4. Love CC. Relationship between sperm motility, morphology and the fertility of stallions. Theriogenology 2011;76:547–57.
5. Jasko DJ, Lein DH, Foote RH. Determination of the relationship between sperm morphologic classifications and fertility in stallions: 66 cases (1987-1988). J Am Vet Med Assoc 1990;197:389–94.
6. Love CC, Varner DD, Thompson JA. Intra- and inter-stallion variation in sperm morphology and their relationship with fertility. J Reprod Fertil Suppl 2000;56: 93–100.
7. Love CC, Noble JK, Standridge SA, et al. The relationship between sperm quality in cool-shipped semen and embryo recovery rate in horses. Theriogenology 2015;84:1587–93.
8. Evenson DP, Darzynkiewicz Z, Melamed MR. Relation of mammalian sperm chromatin heterogeneity to fertility. Science 1980;210:1131.
9. Love CC, Kenney RM. The relationship of increased susceptibility of sperm DNA to denaturation and fertility in the stallion. Theriogenology 1998;50:955–72.
10. Love CC, Thompson JA, Lowry VK, et al. Effect of storage time and temperature on sperm DNA and fertility. Theriogenology 2002;57:1135–42.
11. Henderson SV, Capewell V, Johnson W. Foal registration: transported versus non-transported semen. In: Proceedings 44th Annual American Association of Equine Practitioners. 1998. p. 7–11.
12. Brinkerhoff JM, Love CC, Thompson JA, et al. Influence of mare age, pre-breeding mare status, breeding methods, and stallion on first cycle pregnancy rates on a large commercial breeding farm. Anim Reprod Sci 2010;121:159.
13. Love CC, Brinsko SP, Rigby SL, et al. Relationship of seminal plasma level and extender type to sperm motility and DNA integrity. Theriogenology 2005;63: 1584–91.
14. Kiser AM, Sudderth AK, Love CC, et al. Sperm quality following 4 days of cooled storage: impact on fertility. J Equine Vet Sci 2012;32:491.
15. Jasko DJ, Little TV, Lein DH, et al. Comparison of spermatozoa movement and semen characteristics with fertility in stallions: 64 cases (1987-1988). J Am Vet Med Assoc 1992;200:979–85.
16. Raudsepp T, McCue ME, Das PJ, et al. Genome-wide association study implicates testis-sperm specific FKBP6 as a susceptibility locus for impaired acrosome reaction in stallions. PLoS Genet 2012;8(12):e1003139.
17. Varner DD, Brinsko SP, Blanchard TL, et al. Subfertility in Stallions Associated with Spermatozoal Acrosome Dysfunction. In: Proceedings 47th Annual American Association of Equine Practitioners. 2001. p. 227–8.

Strategies for Processing Semen from Subfertile Stallions for Cooled Transport

Dickson D. Varner, DVM, MS

KEYWORDS

- Equine • Stallion • Semen • Processing • Centrifugation

KEY POINTS

- Simple dilution of semen in extender is generally satisfactory for cooled transport of semen if certain guidelines are applied.
- Subfertility following insemination with cool-transported semen can be associated with different inciting factors.
- Concentration of sperm in semen can be achieved by filtration or centrifugation procedures. Currently, centrifugation is most commonly applied.
- Centrifugal fractionation of semen (also termed density gradient centrifugation) can be used to enhance sperm quality but recovery rates can be low, thereby necessitating low-dose insemination techniques for breeding purposes.

GENERAL GUIDELINES FOR CENTRIFUGATION OF SEMEN

A variety of centrifuge types can be used for centrifugation of semen; however, it is generally recommended to centrifuge semen in a centrifuge fitted with a swinging rotor so that the tubes are held in a horizontal position during the centrifugation process (**Fig. 1**). It is also sensible to secure a centrifuge with adapters that can accommodate either 50-mL or 15-mL centrifuge tubes. Centrifuges come in all shapes and sizes, and rotor radiuses (radii) can vary considerably among these units. Centrifugation speeds can be standardized for all centrifuges by using relative centrifugal force (or gravitational force [g]) to normalize centrifugation speeds among instruments, as opposed to revolutions per minute (RPM). Conversion tables are available for this purpose, as are Web-based conversion programs. Conversions can also be manually calculated

by the following formula: $RPM = \sqrt{\left(\frac{g}{0.0000112 \times r}\right)}$, in which g = relative centrifugal force

Portions of this article were published previously in the *Proceedings of the American Association of Equine Practitioners* and the *Journal of Equine Veterinary Science*.
Department of Large Animal Clinical Sciences, College of Veterinary Medicine and Biomedical Sciences, Texas A&M University, 500 Raymond Stotzer Parkway, College Station, TX 77843-4475, USA
E-mail address: dvarner@cvm.tamu.edu

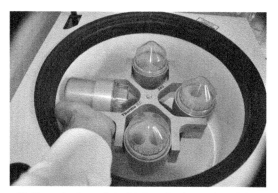

Fig. 1. Centrifuge with the adapter rotated into a horizontal position to demonstrate the mechanics of a swinging rotor during centrifugation. The rotational radius of the rotor can also be determined by measuring from the center of the rotor attachment to the bottom of the adapter when it is held in a horizontal position.

and r = rotational radius (in cm). Therefore, if a centrifuge rotor has a rotational radius of 15.5 cm and the centrifuge speed is designated to be 1000 × g, one would solve for RPM as follows:

$$RPM = \sqrt{\left(\frac{1000}{[0.0000112 \times 15.5]}\right)}$$

$$= \sqrt{\left(\frac{1000}{[0.0001736]}\right)}$$

$$= \sqrt{5760368.664}$$

$$= 2400$$

CUSHIONED CENTRIFUGATION OF SEMEN

As construed from the general principles previously noted for processing semen, concentrating sperm in samples to be prepared for cooled shipment may be necessary to meet the criteria of for maximum seminal plasma concentration (20%) and minimum sperm concentration (25×10^6/mL). This can be achieved by filtration to separate sperm from seminal plasma in raw or extended semen, or by centrifugation of extended semen. Currently, centrifugation of semen is the most commonly applied technique for this purpose. The goal of centrifugation is to maximize sperm recovery rate while avoiding injury to sperm during the centrifugation process. Understandably, an increase in centrifugation time and/or g-force yields an increased sperm recovery rate but it can also lead to decreased sperm quality associated with the amplified mechanical forces of centrifugation and excessive packing of the sperm. Under ideal circumstances, centrifugation would result in a 100% sperm recovery rate with no resulting damage in sperm quality. A variety of centrifugal times and forces have been applied in an attempt to achieve this goal; however, these protocols often lead to a 15% to 20% loss in sperm numbers that could otherwise be used for breeding purposes.

In recent years, a cushioned centrifugation procedure has been applied to stallion semen to maximize sperm harvest without attendant injury to sperm. A nonionic iodinated compound, iodixanol, was first reported for density-gradient somatic cell fractionation, and has since been used as a cushion for centrifugation of sperm. Studies have verified that cushioned centrifugation of stallion semen provides excellent sperm yields of sperm with no attendant sperm damage.[1]

For cushioned centrifugation of sperm, the extended semen is typically loaded in a large-capacity (50 mL) conical-bottom tube, and then a small volume of iodixanol solution is layered beneath the extended semen. The amount of iodixanol solution used for this purpose varies with the laboratory and can be tailored to individual stallions; volumes of 1 to 3.5 mL have been used for this purpose.[2] In instances in which sperm packing is excessive following cushioned centrifugation, the larger volume of cushion fluid provides for a larger surface area for sperm to congregate to minimize this problem. To prepare the tube for centrifugation, extended semen is first placed in the tube and then the cushion fluid is layered beneath the extended semen using an all-plastic syringe attached to a disposable open-end tom cat catheter (3.5 French) or nonbeveled 18-gauge spinal needle (**Figs. 2** and **3**). Following centrifugation, most of the cushion fluid is removed by aspiration. Centrifugation is performed in a centrifuge fitted with a swinging rotor. If iodixanol is used to provide a cushion for centrifugation, semen can be centrifuged at $1000 \times g$ for 20 minutes, yielding a sperm recovery rate approaching 100%, with no apparent injury to the sperm.

When ejaculates contain a low sperm number (eg, $<2 \times 10^9$) and/or sperm concentration is low (eg, $<50 \times 10^6$/mL), it may be prudent to use a modified centrifuge tube, termed a glass nipple-bottom or nipple tube (**Fig. 4**) for centrifugation of semen. These tubes ease the capture of sperm in the postcentrifugation pellet for dilute semen samples while maintaining a high concentration of sperm in the resuspended sample. For this procedure, the nipple portion of the tube is loaded with extender or extended semen (**Fig. 5**) and then 30 μL of iodixanol-based cushion fluid is layered beneath the sample, using a positive displacement pipette (**Fig. 6**). The remainder of the semen and extender can then be added to the tube without disrupting the cushion fluid. The semen is centrifuged at $400 \times g$ for 20 minutes before aspiration of the supernatant (**Fig. 7**). There is no need to remove the cushion fluid before resuspending the sperm pellet. These centrifuge tubes are reusable but require critical cleaning and sterilization between uses (**Fig. 8**). It is also advisable to use siliconized glassware to minimize

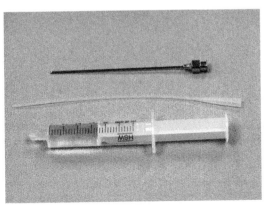

Fig. 2. Cushion fluid can be layered beneath semen before centrifugation by loading in all-plastic syringe and then dispensing through nonbeveled spinal needle or tom cat catheter.

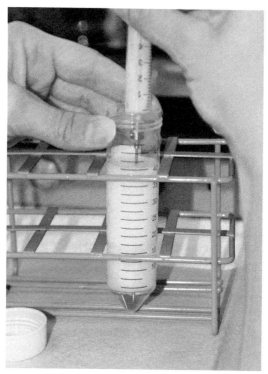

Fig. 3. Dispensing cushion fluid underneath extended semen before centrifugation. Note that the optically clear cushion fluid is easily distinguished from the overlying extended semen.

sperm adherence to the glass. A specially designed centrifuge carrier (adapter) is recommended for this tube type because the nipple portion of the tube is susceptible to breakage if it does not fit properly in the adapter. It is also important to adjust the weight of the filled nipple tube or carrier units before centrifugation (**Fig. 9**). The nipple tubes are manually glass blown so their weights differ and can result in imbalance of the centrifuge if this step is not followed.

Cushioned centrifugation of stallion semen in either conical-bottom tubes containing 1 to 3 mL of iodixanol solution as a cushion or nipple-bottom tubes containing 30 μL of iodixanol solution as a cushion can yield a high sperm harvest while maintaining sperm function. Additionally, an optically opaque extender, as is typically used in the equine breeding industry, can be used to achieve this goal.

GRADIENT CENTRIFUGATION OF SEMEN

Both continuous and discontinuous density centrifugation gradients have been used to separate various cell types in the research laboratory. Continuous centrifugation gradients may be more sensitive for cell selection than discontinuous density gradients but discontinuous gradients are useful when separating cell types with known densities, such as sperm. Application of discontinuous density centrifugation gradients for sperm selection has had broad clinical application in recent years because these gradient procedures are relatively simple to perform and have been shown to effectively separate sperm with various morphologic features in an ejaculate.

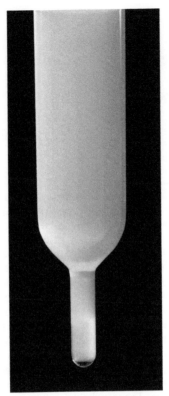

Fig. 4. Glass nipple-bottom tube that can be used to aid in concentrating sperm in dilute ejaculates. Note the sperm pellet contained in the nipple following centrifugation, as well as the small amount of clear cushion fluid underlying the sperm pellet.

Using different concentrations of colloidal silica particles to form density gradients, cells are separated by specific gravity into different layers, based on isopycnic point. Density gradients are advantageous over other methods of sperm separation because the media does not penetrate cell membranes, avoiding potential toxicity. Further,

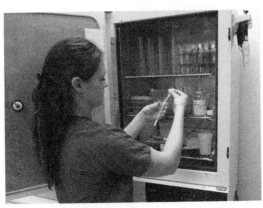

Fig. 5. The nipple portion of the tube is filled with extender or extended semen before added cushion fluid.

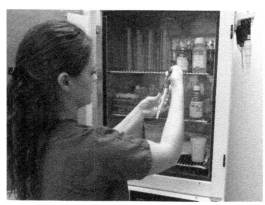

Fig. 6. A small volume (30 μL) of cushion fluid is loaded beneath extender using a positive-displacement pipette with which disposable tips are available.

colloidal silica does not osmotically stress sperm when added to culture medium, it can be formulated into a high specific-gravity to separate dense cells, and it has a low viscosity so as to not impede sperm cell sedimentation. The most well-known discontinuous density gradient, commercialized as Percoll, contains colloidal silica particles coated with polyvinylpyrrolidone. Polyvinylpyrrolidone coating is used to protect cells from the potentially toxic actions of colloidal silica. Percoll was the most widely used discontinuous density gradient in clinical reproductive medicine until the mid-1990s when reports of endotoxin contamination led to removal of this product for clinical use. As a result, alternative discontinuous gradient solutions containing colloidal siliconized silica particles (PureSperm and ISolate) have been used for clinical application with human sperm. These colloidal solutions with siliconized silica particles have been used clinically with human sperm with success comparable to Percoll, and similar products are now being used with stallion sperm.

Centrifugation of equine semen through silanated (or other coated) silica-particle solutions has shown promise for isolating sperm with significantly improved motility,

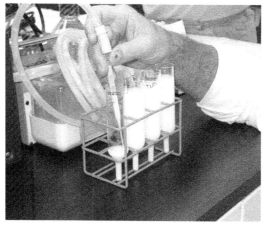

Fig. 7. A vacuum pump is recommended for aspiration of the supernatant because it eliminates the possibility of pellet disruption created by positive pressure (back flow) created within the sample.

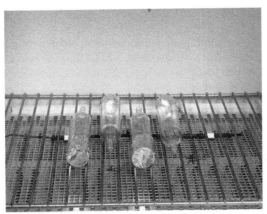

Fig. 8. Glass nipple bottom tubes can be covered with aluminum foil after cleaning and drying, then placed in oven (100°C) for 30 minutes to sterilize before use.

morphology, and chromatin quality, and enhancing the fertility of selected subfertile stallions.[3,4] The author's laboratory has found that sperm recovery rate is higher, when using 15-mL capacity conical-bottom tubes, compared with 50-mL capacity conical-bottom tubes for this purpose; that use of a 1-layer gradient yields a higher sperm recovery rate than a 2-layer gradient; and that gradient volumes of 2, 3, or

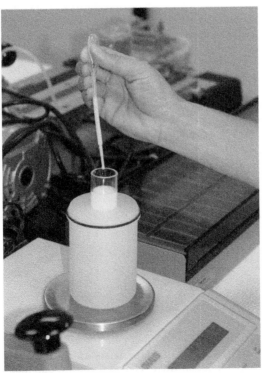

Fig. 9. It is important to adjust the weights of loaded nipple-bottom tubes by adding additional extender so that all are the same weight before centrifugation.

4 mL in 15-mL centrifugation tubes yield similar semen quality and sperm recovery rates.[3]

When using gradient centrifugation (also termed centrifugal fractionation) to optimize sperm quality, the laboratory generally applies this centrifugation method after first subjecting the semen to cushioned centrifugation (as previously described) to increase the sperm concentration in the sample to 300 to 500 $\times$ 10^6/mL. The concentrated sample is then gently layered over the silica particle solution with a maximum of 500 $\times$ 10^6 sperm applied over gradient solution in each 15-mL tube (**Figs. 10** and **11**). The loaded tubes are then subjected to centrifugation at 200 $\times$ g for 30 min. Following centrifugation, all supernate above the sperm pellet is aspirated and the sperm are resuspended in a small volume of extender such that the resulting product contains 100 to 300 $\times$ 10^6 sperm/mL for insemination purposes. Sperm harvest following gradient centrifugation varies widely among stallions and depends, in large part, on the sperm quality, that is, the sperm morphologic profile of the ejaculate. Recovery rates of 20% to 30% are not uncommon in stallions with a high percentages of certain sperm morphologic defects, such as abnormally large heads, abnormally shaped midpieces, bent tails, and coiled tails, because these sperm are largely removed during the centrifugation or sperm resuspension procedure. Owing to the relatively low sperm recovery rates that are generally achieved following gradient centrifugation of semen with reduced quality, low-dose insemination procedures are generally needed for breeding purposes.

LOW-DOSE INSEMINATION

The threshold number of sperm that can be used to inseminate mares and yield a high pregnancy rate is highly variable but this number is certainly affected by the fertility of a given stallion and by the semen processing method that is applied (eg, cooled storage or cryopreservation) before insemination. Using customary methods, mares are inseminated with 250 million to 1 billion progressively motile sperm in a volume of 10 to 50 mL deposited directly into the lumen of the uterine body. The laboratory has reported that, surprisingly, less than 0.0007% of sperm that are deposited into mare uteri actually gain access into the oviducts. However, insemination in the tip of the uterine horn ipsilateral to an ovary containing a dominant follicle resulted in a

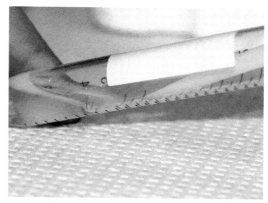

Fig. 10. For centrifugal fractionation of sperm, extended semen can be gently layered over the colloidal silica particle solution while holding the centrifuge tube at an acute angle. Care should be taken to create a distinct interface between the gradient solution and the overlying semen.

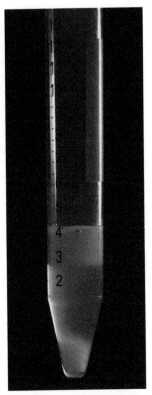

Fig. 11. Centrifugation of sperm through a density gradient yields a distinctive sperm pellet. If ejaculate (case) selection is proper, the sperm pellet generally contains a disproportionately higher percentage of sperm with improved morphology, motility, and chromatin quality.

greater percentage of oviductal sperm (77%) recovered from the ipsilateral oviduct, compared with uterine body insemination (54%).[5] These data indicate that more sperm gain access into the oviduct of fertilization when the insemination location is the tip of the uterine horn as opposed to the uterine body.

This breeding technique, termed deep-uterine low-dose insemination, has been examined in the research setting, and applied clinically in recent years. Two techniques are most commonly used for deposition of an insemination dose on or near the oviductal papilla: (1) use of a video-endoscope (termed hysteroscope) to visually locate the papilla and permit accurate placement of semen via a long catheter passed through the biopsy channel of the insertion tube and (2) use of a flexible catheter (usually double-lumen) in which the catheter tip is guided to a position adjacent to the papilla by manipulation per rectum before deposition of semen. The optimal method for low-dose insemination of mares is subject to debate. Recent findings in the laboratory revealed no difference between the 2 methods when mares were inseminated with as little as 0.5 to 1×10^6 sperm from a stallion with known good fertility.[6] Certainly, the hysteroscopic technique has the disadvantages of increased equipment costs, an increased labor force, and increased time for insemination. As such, the transrectally guided approach would seem to lend itself more favorably to widespread application in the equine breeding industry. Heighted skill of the attending veterinarian, however, is necessary for this latter technique to be successful.

Clinical Case 1

A 12-year-old quarter horse was admitted to the Texas Veterinary Medical Center for assessment of fertility and to determine if altered strategies of breeding management could improve pregnancy rates. According to the owner, the stallion had been fertile in previous years but per-cycle pregnancy rate dropped to approximately 35% in the previous season when covering approximately 90 mares. Total testicular volume of this stallion was calculated to be 184 mL. Predicted daily sperm output (DSO), as determined from testicular volume, was 3.7×10^9 sperm but actual DSO was approximately 1.7×10^9 sperm; therefore, spermatogenic efficiency was estimated to be less than 50%. Ejaculates contained an average of 33% morphologically normal sperm and 38% progressively motile sperm. The most common morphologic defects were bent tails (average of 35%) and abnormally shaped midpieces (average of 33%). The average percentage of progressively motile sperm following 24 hours of cooled storage of extended semen was 29%.

Centrifugation of extended semen was proposed as a means to increase sperm concentration in inseminates because sperm concentration in raw ejaculates was generally less than 100×10^6 per mL (range of 28–109×10^6/mL, median of 68×10^6/mL). Extended semen from the stallion was subjected to cushioned centrifugation for 20 min at $400 \times g$, using glass nipple-bottom centrifuge tubes to reduce seminal plasma concentration and increase sperm concentration in resuspended sperm pellets. Reproductively normal mares were inseminated with processed semen to evaluate the effects of sperm number, storage time, and insemination method on fertility. Owing to the costs associated with a breeding trial, the client was amenable only to insemination of a small group of mares to determine if simple concentration of sperm and transrectally guided or hysteroscopic low-dose insemination techniques would result in pregnancy rates that would allow this stallion to be commercially viable (**Table 1**).

Although the number of mares inseminated in each of the 5 treatment groups was small, the outcome was sufficient to provide generalizations regarding treatment strategies for the subject stallion. The results suggest that no difference in fertility existed between inseminates of 250×10^6 or 500×10^6 total sperm. Cooled storage of semen had no apparent deleterious effect on fertility, and transrectally guided insemination of semen yielded results that were similar to, or exceeded, that of hysteroscopic insemination. A follow-up trial with cool-transported semen resulted in recovery and transfer of 5 embryos from 4 mares inseminated.

Table 1
Effects of sperm number, insemination volume, and method of insemination on pregnancy rate in mares, with semen from a single stallion

Total Sperm in Inseminate ($\times 10^6$)	Storage Time for Processed Semen (h)	Volume of Inseminate (mL)	Method of Insemination	Per-cycle Pregnancy Rate (%)
500	0	1	Transrectally guided	4/6 (66%)
500	24	1	Transrectally guided	4/6 (66%)
250	0	0.5	Transrectally guided	5/6 (83%)
250	24	0.5	Transrectally guided	4/6 (66%)
250	0	0.2	Hysteroscopic	1/2 (50%)

Semen from this stallion had not previously been subjected to cooled storage and transport. The stallion was discharged with recommendations to use cushioned centrifugation of semen and transrectally guided insemination with 250 million sperm per mare initially, with the prospect that sperm number in inseminates could be lowered if initial pregnancy results were favorable. In addition, the owner was informed of the potential value of cool-stored semen. A decision was made to breed mares the following season primarily with fresh processed semen. A total of 132 mares were bred over 170 cycles, with cool-transported semen used on only 3 occasions. The stallion achieved a seasonal pregnancy rate of 85% with an average of 1.5 cycles per pregnancy (ie, a per-cycle pregnancy rate of 66%).

Clinical Case 2

A 6-year-old quarter horse stallion was admitted to the Texas Veterinary Medical Center for a breeding soundness examination and for potential therapeutic approaches to improve his fertility. The stallion was administered an orally active progestogen, altrenogest (Regu-Mate, Intervet/Schering-Plough Animal Health, Millsboro, Delaware, USA), on a daily basis during his 4-year athletic career. The dosage of altrenogest administered was unknown to the owner of the stallion. Only 1 mare was pregnant from the first 8 mares inseminated with entire ejaculates, resulting in a 12% per-cycle pregnancy rate.

The stallion had a total testicular volume of 134 mL and a predicted DSO, based on testicular volume, of 2.5×10^9 sperm. Actual DSO for the stallion was approximately 1×10^9 sperm, so spermatogenic efficiency was determined to less than 50%. Ejaculates contained an average of 15% morphologically normal sperm and 34% progressively motile sperm. The most common sperm morphologic defects were abnormally shaped midpieces (average of 28%) and bent tails (average of 22%).

After consultation with the owner, a decision was made to inseminate a small group of reproductively normal mares by low-dose insemination techniques. Semen-processing techniques consisted of cushioned centrifugation only or cushioned centrifugation followed by density-gradient centrifugation through a silanated silica-particle solution. The density-gradient centrifugation procedure was used in an attempt to improve semen quality through separation of spermatozoal morphologic types based on isopycnic point. Results of the clinical trial are provided in **Table 2**.

Pregnancy rates improved as insemination dose increased from 15 to 100×10^6 progressively motile sperm, indicating a dose-dependent effect of insemination number on fertility. Following cushioned centrifugation, no distinct advantage was gained by using hysteroscopic insemination, compared with transrectally-guided insemination in the tip of the uterine horn. Insemination in the tip of the uterine horn, however, yielded a higher pregnancy rate than standard insemination in the uterine body when the inseminate contained 100×10^6 progressively motile sperm. Further processing of semen through a silica particle solution also seemed to improve pregnancy rates, in comparison with only cushioned centrifugation, when the inseminate contained 50×10^6 progressively motile sperm.

The stallion was discharged from the hospital with instructions to breed mares with a low-dose insemination technique, using a minimum of 100×10^6 progressively motile sperm following cushioned centrifugation or 50×10^6 progressively motile sperm following gradient centrifugation. The author also proposed that the insemination dose with semen treated by gradient centrifugation might be lowered, without negatively affecting fertility but that this possibility should be tested before it could be recommended for commercial purposes. The fertility of cool-stored semen was not tested so recommendations regarding its use could not be offered. The owner

Table 2
Effects of semen-processing technique, method of insemination, and number of progressively motile sperm in inseminates on pregnancy rate in mares, with semen from a single stallion

Centrifugation Technique	Method of Insemination	Progressively Motile Sperm in Inseminate ($\times 10^6$)	Inseminate Volume (mL)	Per-cycle Pregnancy Rate (%)
Cushioned method	Transrectally guided	15	1	0/6 (0%)
Cushioned method	Transrectally guided	50	1	2/6 (33%)
Cushioned method	Transrectally guided	100	1	5/6 (83%)
Cushioned method	Hysteroscopic	50	0.1	3/8 (38%)
Cushioned method	Standard uterine body	100	1	2/6 (33%)
Density gradient	Hysteroscopic	50	0.1	6/8 (75%)

indicated that the stallion had normal fertility the following breeding season when mares were inseminated by a transrectally guided technique using semen previously subjected to cushioned centrifugation. The precise mare book, insemination doses, and fertility statistics were not available.

Clinical Case 3

A 4-year-old quarter horse stallion was admitted to the Texas Veterinary Medical Center for evaluation of breeding soundness following his first season at stud during which he achieved a 59% seasonal pregnancy rate when covering 165 mares. Approximately one-half of the mares were bred with cool-transported semen. During that breeding season, progressive sperm motility was estimated to be 70% for 76 of the 84 semen collections performed and the average total sperm number in the 84 ejaculates was approximately 5.349×10^9 sperm. The sperm concentration was estimated to be less than 100×10^6 sperm/mL for 67 of the 84 ejaculates collected.

The testicular volume of this stallion was determined to be 225 mL, resulting in a predicted DSO of 4.6×10^9 sperm, assuming the testes were producing sperm with normal efficiency. Four ejaculates were collected from the stallion. The stallion's actual sperm output on the fourth daily collection was 3.67×10^9 sperm, so spermatogenic efficiency was considered to be below normal. The percentage of morphologically normal sperm in ejaculates averaged 38%, and the percentage of progressively motile sperm averaged 27%. The most common morphologic defects were abnormally shaped midpieces (average of 30%) and bent tails (19%).

Semen from 3 ejaculates was processed by cushioned centrifugation alone or by cushioned centrifugation followed by gradient centrifugation. Semen was evaluated for sperm motility immediately following each processing step and following 24 hours of cooled storage. The effect of seminal plasma was also evaluated. The semen morphologic profiles of unprocessed (raw) semen and semen subjected to gradient centrifugation were also compared. Data from a representative ejaculate are provided in **Tables 3** and **4**.

From these data, one can surmise that the gradient centrifugation procedure considerably improved the semen quality of this stallion because measures of sperm

Table 3
Effects of semen processing protocol (simple dilution, cushioned centrifugation, or density gradient centrifugation), source of seminal plasma (same stallion or fertile control stallion), and storage time (0 or 24 h) on measures of sperm motility

Centrifugation Technique	Source of Seminal Plasma	Sperm Concentration ($\times 10^6$/ml)	Storage Time (h)	Total Motility (%)	Progressive Motility (%)	Curvilinear Velocity (μm/s)
Simple dilution	Same	30	0	54	21	176
Cushioned centrifugation	Same	30	0	59	33	121
Density gradient	Same	30	0	90	77	146
Density gradient	Control	30	0	93	82	224
Simple dilution	Same	30	24	50	20	136
Cushioned centrifugation	Same	200	24	59	29	152
Cushioned centrifugation	Same	30	24	56	33	135
Density gradient	Same	200	24	87	72	141
Density gradient	Control	200	24	89	73	208

motility and sperm morphology were enhanced with this procedure. The increase in the percentage of morphologically normal sperm following gradient centrifugation was primarily attributable to reduced percentages of abnormal (irregular or bent) mid-pieces, and bent tails. For this ejaculate, and others evaluated from this stallion, sperm velocity was increased when seminal plasma from the test stallion was replaced with that obtained a fertile control stallion. For all treatments in **Table 3**, sperm motility values did not change appreciably following 24 hours of cooled storage, compared with that evaluated before storage.

A follow-up fertility trial was conducted with semen from this stallion to determine if insemination of mares with semen subjected to gradient centrifugation would improve

Table 4
Effect of semen centrifugation through density gradient solution on sperm morphologic features, as viewed by differential-interference microscopy at 1250 × magnification

Sperm Morphologic Feature (%)	Unprocessed (Raw) Semen	Density Gradient Processed Semen
Normal	40	76
Abnormal heads	5	1
Abnormal acrosomes	1	1
Tailless heads	3	2
Proximal protoplasmic droplets	10	5
Distal protoplasmic droplets	13	5
Abnormal (irregular) midpieces	28	6
Bent midpieces	13	3
Bent tails	19	5
Coiled tails	1	0
Premature (round) germ cells	1	0

pregnancy rates. Ten reproductively normal mares were inseminated in this trial; each of 5 mares was inseminated once with 100×10^6 total sperm and each of 5 mares was inseminated once with 200×10^6 total sperm. The test stallion's seminal plasma was replaced with that of a fertile donor stallion. Seminal plasma from donor was procured by centrifuging raw semen for $1000 \times g$ for 15 minutes, followed by filtration of supernate through tandem 5.0- and 1.2-micron pore-size nylon filters to remove any remaining sperm from the seminal plasma. One-ml aliquots of seminal plasma were frozen in vials at -80°C before use. Inseminate volumes ranged from 0.25 to 0.58 mL and a transrectally guided low-dose insemination technique was used. The per-cycle pregnancy rates were 100% (5/5) for mares inseminated with 100×10^6 total sperm, and 4 out of 5 (80%) for mares inseminated with 200×10^6 total sperm. Two mares, 1 in each treatment group, experienced double ovulations, and each of these mares was diagnosed with twin pregnancies. As such, pregnancy rate per ovulation was 100% (6 out of 6) for mares inseminated with 100×10^6 total sperm, and 5 out of 6 (83%) for mares inseminated with 200×10^6 total sperm. Based on the postcentrifugation recovery rate of sperm in this trial, the stallion would have had sufficient semen to breed 17 mares per ejaculate if mares were to be inseminated with 100×10^6 total sperm.

For the following commercial breeding season, 212 mares were inseminated, primarily using fresh density-gradient-treated semen with seminal plasma from a fertile donor stallion. The stallion achieved a seasonal pregnancy rate of 91% in an average of 1.61 cycles per pregnancy (ie, a per-cycle pregnancy rate of 62%).

SUMMARY

Equine veterinarians may encounter owners of stallions who are seeking methods that can improve stallion breeding performance. Breeding and semen-manipulation strategies can be applied to maximize the fertility of these stallions and to extend their productive life. Any recommended breeding modifications can often be tested outside the commercial breeding season by conducting clinical fertility trials. Recipient-mare herds retained by embryo-transfer facilities are an excellent source for such trials. The information gained provides useful information for the stallion owner or agent preparing for a forthcoming breeding season.

REFERENCES

1. Waite JA, Love CC, Brinsko SP, et al. Factors impacting equine sperm recovery rate and quality following cushioned centrifugation. Theriogenology 2008;70: 704–14.
2. Bliss SB, Voge JL, Hayden SS, et al. The impact of cushioned centrifugation protocols on semen quality. Theriogenology 2012;77:1232–9.
3. Edmond AJ, Brinsko SP, Love CC, et al. Effect of centrifugal fractionation protocols on quality and recovery rate of equine sperm. Theriogenology 2012;77:959–66.
4. Varner DD, Love CC, Brinsko SP, et al. Semen processing for the subfertile stallion. J Equine Vet Sci 2008;28:677–85.
5. Rigby S, Derczo S, Brinsko S, et al. Oviductal sperm numbers following proximal uterine horn or uterine body insemination. Proc Am Assoc Equine Pract 2000;46: 332–4.
6. Hayden SS, Blanchard TL, Brinsko SP, et al. Pregnancy rates in mares inseminated with 0.5 or 1 million sperm using hysteroscopic or transrectally guided deep-horn insemination techniques. Theriogenology 2012;78:914–20.

Index

Note: Page numbers of article titles are in **boldface** type.

Vet Clin Equine 32 (2016) 561–570
http://dx.doi.org/10.1016/S0749-0739(16)30060-8
0749-0739/16/$ – see front matter

Moving?

Make sure your subscription moves with you!

To notify us of your new address, find your **Clinics Account Number** (located on your mailing label above your name), and contact customer service at:

Email: journalscustomerservice-usa@elsevier.com

800-654-2452 (subscribers in the U.S. & Canada)
314-447-8871 (subscribers outside of the U.S. & Canada)

Fax number: 314-447-8029

Elsevier Health Sciences Division
Subscription Customer Service
3251 Riverport Lane
Maryland Heights, MO 63043

*To ensure uninterrupted delivery of your subscription, please notify us at least 4 weeks in advance of move.